Nikki Bradford is an award-winning author and medical journalist. She has written 10 health books, some of which have been translated into 12 languages and sold world-wide, including *The Miraculous World of Your Unborn Baby* (1998), *What They Don't Tell You About Being a Mother and Having Babies* (1997), *The Hamlyn Encyclopaedia of Complementary Health* (1996) and *Men's Health Matters – the Ultimate Guide to Male Bodies* (1995). She was formerly Health Correspondent for *Good Housekeeping* magazine, Health Editor on *Essentials*, and founding Honorary Secretary for The Guild of Health Writers. She lives by the seaside in Sussex, has two young children, Ben and Jessie, three cats and a part-share in a boa constrictor called Diamond Lil.

Also available in Orion paperback

APPLES & PEARS
Gloria Thomas

ARE YOU GETTING ENOUGH?
Angela Dowden

AROUSING AROMAS
Kay Cooper

COPING WITH YOUR PREMATURE BABY
Dr Penny Stanway

EAT SAFELY
Janet Wright

FIRST BABY AFTER THIRTY ... OR FORTY?
Dr Penny Stanway

THE GOOD MOOD GUIDE
Ros & Jeremy Holmes

HARMONISE YOUR HOME
Graham Gunn

HEALTH SPA AT HOME
Josephine Fairley

JUICE UP YOUR ENERGY LEVELS
Lesley Waters

SENSITIVE SKIN
Josephine Fairley

SPRING CLEAN YOUR SYSTEM
Jane Garton

NATURAL PAINKILLERS

NIKKI BRADFORD

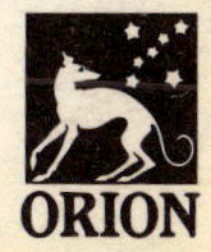

An Orion Paperback
First published in Great Britain in 1999 by
Orion Books Ltd,
Orion House, 5 Upper St Martin's Lane,
London WC2H 9EA

A CIP catalogue record for this book
is available from the British Library.

ISBN: 0 75281 603 9

Printed and bound in Great Britain by
The Guernsey Press Co. Ltd, Guernsey, C.I.

CONTENTS

ACKNOWLEDGMENTS

With very grateful thanks to three very exceptional practitioners, whose advice and help has been invaluable for this little book:

Dr Shreyas Patel, consultant neurologist and pain treatment specialist
Shreyas is Consultant Neurologist and Medical Director of the Pain & Stress Reduction Programs at The Marino Center for Progressive Health in Cambridge, Massachusetts, USA. He is also Consultant Neurologist at St Elisabeth's Hospital Medical Center, Boston, and former lecturer at Harvard Medical School.

Farah Begum-Baig, reflexologist and research scientist
Farah was a research scientist at Cambridge University in England, and is now Director of the Hope Clinic, a leading complementary medicine centre in Cambridge, England. She has been a major force in pioneering the use of complementary therapies within the NHS in Britain, and teaches reflexology for stress reduction and obstetric purposes to doctors, nurses and midwives at Addenbrookes Hospital and Ely Hospital in Cambridgeshire. Farah has contributed to several books on complementary medicine, and regularly appears on national TV and radio.

Phillip Beech, osteopath, naturopath and acupuncturist
Phillip runs his own top osteopathy, naturopathy and acupuncture practice in Hampstead, London. He also lectures and teaches at the British College of Naturopathy and Osteopathy, and the British School of Osteopathy (both in London) and has a special interest in how eastern forms of healing treatments such as acupuncture can be translated into the framework of western medicine.

INTRODUCTION

What this book can do for you

'Prolonged pain has the power to crush our self-confidence and lead us to lose our sense of who we are. It is rather like being trapped in an endlessly revolving door… This brings us to the first lesson of pain relief, and it may come as a surprise: the only effective way to overcome pain is to do something about it ourselves.'

Dr Chris Wells, past director of the pioneering Centre for Pain Relief, Walton Hospital, Liverpool.

Doing something about it for ourselves – not asking a doctor to prescribe it or a nurse to administer it – is what this little book is all about. For every type of pain you may feel there is always something out there that you can do to help yourself to soothe or alleviate it – maybe a little, but maybe a lot. The problem is knowing what your options are, and finding the right one for you. This is also what *Natural Painkillers* is all about.

This self-help approach is not meant to replace medical treatment from a qualified practitioner. It is meant to back it up, to complement it, to keep you going until your medicine kicks in, and – to paraphrase the Holstein Pils advertisment – to reach some of the parts that ordinary medical treatment cannot reach. Tincture of echinacea on a screaming toothache can hold it until you can get to your dentist. Burning cystitis? A combination of litres of diluted lemon barley and peeing under the shower could see you through. A raging, ground-glass sore throat? Gargle with red sage tea – it's as good as a local anaesthetic. Your child has fallen and a really painful great bruise is coming up? Gently rubbing on arnica cream or applying a cool compress of the herb rosemary will soothe the throb. And if the pain of severe rheumatoid arthritis or back disc degeneration responds to nothing else, cannabis painkilling tea has, anecdotally, helped many (see p. 32).

This self-help approach is not meant to replace medical treatment from a qualified practitioner

All these and many, many more options which you can do for yourself can play a really vital role whether the pain you have is short- or long-term, and this book has many practical suggestions which will offer different routes to explore if the help your doctor gives you is not enough. With a chronic (rather than acute) pain, the bad news is that there is no single quick fix. The very good news is, however, that there will very probably be other helpful strategies and therapies you can check out, ones which will attack the problem slowly but surely from different angles until you finally tame it or, better still, it eventually melts away altogether. Either way, you get back some control over your life.

A raging, ground-glass sore throat? Gargle with red sage tea

Natural Painkillers looks through many of the most common types of pain and at what you personally can do about them right now. Because the book is small and the subject so big, it can only give tasters and pointers rather than the Full Monty, but it also lists as many help lines and advisory organisations as possible that can tell you where to find out more as a good jumping-off point. Just as importantly, *Natural Painkillers* also backs up most of the suggestions it makes, with brief details of the published clinical trials and references (see p.146) whether it's black cohosh herb for sharp period pains or homeopathic thuja for prostatitis.

HOW PAIN WORKS

There are two types of pain: acute and chronic. The acute variety is what you feel if you are unlucky enough to drop a concrete block on your foot or burn your hand on the cooker. This type does a very useful job by giving us an unmistakable warning that you are hurt, and it triggers the impetus to do something about it fast – such as snatching your hand back from that cooker. Acute pain is protective, positive – and it goes away after a while.

Chronic pain doesn't go away and can have many different causes – such as osteoporosis, rheumatoid arthritis or an injury. It does not serve any useful practical purpose, and may be hard, or downright impossible, to treat. Often the amount you feel seems to be bafflingly out of proportion to its physical cause. This in no way suggests that you are imagining it. Far from it.

What chronic pain does mean – and doctors everywhere now accept this – is that there is a hefty emotional or psychological

Acute pain is protective, positive – and it goes away after a while

factor in it. Our feelings and attitudes towards chronic pain, and our mood, whether deliberately relaxed, determinedly positive or downhearted, can profoundly affect the level of pain you actually register.

This is good news, because it shows us what enormous power the mind of every single one of us has to affect how much pain we feel. Our own mind can therefore be the one transcendentally powerful weapon we can use to fight back.

This is why all good pain units and clinics, such as St Thomas Hospital in London or the Walton in Liverpool, have self-empowerment programmes and relaxation classes for long-term pain sufferers and why they place such emphasis on the self-management of chronic pain. It's why psychologists such as US practitioner Dr Robert Ornstein are such fans of laughter therapy for treating (or warding off) illness and discomfort, or why fashionable private dentists, such as the White Cross chain in London, run continuous MTV inches from their patients upturned faces when getting down to serious drilling. It's also probably why one woman in labour at Guys Hospital in 1989 memorably sang *Ten Green Bottles* 948 times during childbirth. 'It seemed to keep her spirits up and her mind at least partially elsewhere, though the other mothers got a bit tired of it,' commented the then head of obstetrics, Professor Mike Chapman. 'I prefer it when they meditate myself.'

Your mind is elsewhere. Exactly. Pain is a mind/body double act. Positive emotions and distraction act as gates that can partially close some of the nerve pathways to the brain allowing fewer pain messages through to be registered and felt. Yet this same double act will work against us too, given half the chance. Dark emotions such as fear and depression can have a powerful negative effect, as with the vicious circle of long-term severe back trouble and depression.

Dark emotions such as fear and depression can have a powerful negative effect

FAST AND SLOW PAIN

Another factor which affects the level of physical distress you actually register is whether you are experiencing fast, or slow pain.

Fast pain is when you prick your finger and feel a sharp flare of discomfort at the exact spot of injury, which then becomes a slow burning ache (slow pain) in the general area. Fast pain attracts our undivided attention and rapid automatic response. Slow pain is more complicated because the level at which you register it can depend on your state of mind at the time – how tired or stressed you are, on memories of how your parents might have reacted if they did something similar when you were a small child, or even how much you were expecting it to hurt in the first place.

PAIN TOLERANCE AND PAIN THRESHOLDS

'My God – he must have a high pain threshold' people say, as they watch a heavyweight boxer withstanding a hammering round after round in the ring. He hasn't, but the chances are that he may have developed a high pain *tolerance* instead. Or, 'Huh – she had an epidural after the first few contractions – what a pathetically low pain threshold,' says one mum who gave birth using breathing control alone of another who exercised her option of an epidural as soon as possible. Wrong again. It's the two womens' tolerance levels that varied, and you can influence these considerably if you know how. Despite the heavily implied criticism, bravery doesn't come into it.

Though the two terms are often used inaccurately, even interchangeably, pain tolerance is linked to slow pain, and it is the measure of how much discomfort you can take. It varies from person to person, and depends a lot on the circumstances you are in at the time – whether you are relatively cheerful and calm, or a frazzled bundle of terrified foreboding. Pain threshold is different. It is the physiological point at which something begins to hurt. In healthy individuals, everyone's pain thresholds are pretty similar, though they can be affected by illness, tiredness, hunger, even how hot or cold the climate is. If you ask a tester for instance to hold a metal rod which is slowly heating up or being frozen, the ouch point is invariably 43 degrees C or -6 degrees C.

HOW PAIN TRAVELS – AND HOW TO STOP IT

Fast and slow pain signals are transmitted to the brain by networks of nerve endings that are scattered throughout the body, called pain receptors. It is their job to monitor sensations. Both fast and slow pain signals have different types of pathways for carrying pain messages to the brain. The signals take the form of a very small electrical current which passes from cell to cell. Essentially one end of the cell is a receiver that picks up the message, the other end releases chemicals called neurotransmitters.

There are several different varieties of chemicals involved in pain transmission, including Substance P and serotonin. Their job is to help the electrical pain or sensation message jump across the small gap (synapse) between one nerve cell ending and the next. These chemicals are rapidly destroyed after use – they have to be, otherwise our muscles would be permanently twitching – by an enzyme called acetylecholinesterase. This transmission/destruction process may sound laborious but it works at warp speed.

Your body helps you to cope with chronic slow pain by manufacturing its own endorphins

Your body helps you to cope with chronic slow pain by manufacturing its own endorphins, (naturally produced morphine-like chemicals). Slow pain also responds to morphine-based drugs. We also have an inbuilt way of coping way with fast pain – 'gating' or blocking some of the neurological signals to the brain by interfering with their transmission paths. For instance, rubbing a banged knee is done instinctively, but for a very good reason – the pressure and friction reduce the amount of pain messages getting through to the brain so that you feel (register) less discomfort, even though the level of actual tissue damage done at the injured place remains the same.

Much of the advice in this book is based on the above, as well as on natural forms of analgesia such as pain-killing herbs, homeopathic and nutritional medicines. Hopefully you might perhaps find several remedies that you can use – whether it's taking the throb out of varicose veins, soothing pre-period breast pain or calming a vicious earache – without visiting your doctor.

AND FINALLY...THE POWER OF PRAYER AND LAUGHTER

Both are relevant to helping every type of pain, especially the long-term chronic conditions such as backache, arthritis, shingles, IBS and sciatica. They can also be an invaluable aid to reducing the stress that tends to exacerbate these sort of conditions – and most others, come to that, because 'anywhere from sixty to ninety per cent of visits to doctors are in the mind/body stress-related realm' reckons Dr Herbert Benson, president of the Mind/Body Medical Institute of Boston's Deaconess Hospital and Harvard Medical School.

Laughter can physically raise pain tolerance levels, and there are studies to prove it. One American study in 1985 for instance, which had student volunteers listening to twenty minutes of comedienne Lily Tomlin telling Alexander Graham Bell jokes, rendered them far less sensitive to experimental pain stimulus than their friends who were wired up to a breath-takingly dull lecture entitled 'Ethics and the Sociology of Peer Review'. Some researchers speculate that laughter triggers the release of endorphins, others that it is pure distraction therapy.

Laughter can physically raise pain tolerance levels

No one has been able to explain why spiritual healing and prayer can help so much, though they are now becoming sufficiently mainstream to be used in some NHS centres in the UK, such as the Hammersmith Hospital's gold-standard oncology unit under Professor Karel Sikora. Both have been the subject of clinical trials, though assessing prayer power scientifically can be, as Professor William Jarvis of California's Loma Linda University and president of the National Council Against Health Fraud puts it, 'like trying to nail Jell'o to the wall'.

However, one study by San Francisco cardiologist Randolph Byrd at the SF General Hospital discovered something that was hard to put down to a placebo effect. He took 393 coronary care patients and randomly assigned half to be prayed for by born-again Christians. He carefully did not tell his patients who was being prayed for and who wasn't. He found that the group that wasn't needed five times as many antibiotics and were three times as likely to develop complications as the prayer group.

In 1995, Dr Elisabeth Targ, clinical director of Psychosocial Oncology Research at the California Pacific Medical Center arranged for a group of twenty severely ill AIDS patients to test out prayer power too, in that half were prayed for and meditated upon at a distance and half not. Though she has not yet published the precise results, she describes them as encouraging enough to warrant a much bigger follow-up study. If you would like to explore this option further, contact the National Federation of Spiritual Healers, Old Manor Farm Studio, Church Street, Sunbury on Thames TW16 6RG. Tel: 01932 783 164. They can arrange distant healing by prayer and also one-to-one sessions where they come to see you at your home, hospital, hospice, or at a special healing clinic. Some healers charge as much as £15-£35 plus per session, but payment is usually by donation only (around £2-5, plus travel expenses if relevant). If you are ill but do not have any money, there tends to be no charge at all.

THE THERAPIES

Which self-help therapy?

The best thing about pain is that it can be highly responsive to self-help treatments and strategies. With an acute and short-term pain such as a raging toothache or a lacerating sore throat, some well-timed sensible, DIY measures can get you through until you can see someone (a GP or a good, professionally qualified complementary therapist). For recurrent, familiar pain such as period pain (once you have checked with a doctor that there is no underlying cause that needs specific treatment), the coping strategy – whether it's the pain-relieving herb white willow, or gentle yoga stretches and a warm lavender and rose essential oil tummy rub – gives you a good measure of control over the situation. For chronic long-term pain, pain experts say that an integrated self-help plan perhaps incorporating several different elements that you have found work the best for you, may be far more effective than painkilling drugs alone.

Complementary therapies lend themselves to some basic, sensible DIY usage, with the exception of the heavily manipulative therapies such as osteopathy and chiropractic which you cannot do for yourself. In this book I have set out very brief details about what acupressure, aromatherapy, nutritional supplements, homeopathy, herbs, reflexology and visualisation offer, as these can all be very helpful and you can carry out their basic treatments for yourself. It's worth knowing, however, that you will get even better results if you work with a really good, professionally qualified complementary therapist as well as using DIY techniques at home. If you can have expert assessment and monitoring as necessary, plus some good professional treatments and a self-help consultation, DIY treatments will be that much more effective. To find a properly trained practitioner in your area, contact the professional association listed in this chapter.

There are also some traditional doctors (mostly private but a few NHS) who have had training in therapies such as acupressure/ acupuncture, and have full training in homeopathy.

Note: the costs of professional sessions vary widely depending on the experience of the therapist, and where you live.

For published clinical references to any trials mentioned below, see p. 146.

The best thing about pain is that it can be highly responsive to self-help treatments

ACUPRESSURE

Acupressure involves using fingertip or thumb-tip pressure on any of the 365 different acupuncture points around the body. These points have traditional Chinese names, such as Happy Calm, Bright and Clear, and Three Mile Leg, though they are also referred to as numbers (e.g. Liv 3, for point number three on the Liver meridian) and are dotted all over the body's twelve main energy channels, or pathways. Treatments may also include massage along these pathways. Practitioners explain that this stimulates the body's energy flow, or chi. Essentially, acupressure is acupuncture without the needles.

Acupressure has been used in many hundreds of proper clinical trials and usually comes out well. One such trial in 1986 with factory car workers who had chronic lower-back pain resulted in one in five showing 'a marked improvement', and half saying they were completely cured.

Therapist: there is no official body for acupressure therapists. Instead, contact one of the acupuncture organisations (as practitioners are invariably trained in both) such as The British Acupuncture Council, 63 Jeddo Road, London W12 9HQ. Tel: 0181 735 0400.

Approx cost: From £15 to £40 a session.

Acupressure is acupuncture without the needles

AROMATHERAPY

This therapy uses the scented extracts of plants (flowers, herbs, spices and even trees) to promote well-being and a skilled, professional aromatherapist can help treat specific disorders and soothe certain types of pain as well. Essential oils are usually mixed with a carrier oil and massaged on to the body. Though skin is generally an effective barrier, small amounts of the oil (enough to be effective) can reach the bloodstream via the hair and sweat follicles which go down into the dermis (growing layer) of skin, which is fed directly by a rich network of tiny blood capillaries. The oils can also be added to boiling water and inhaled as steam, where again they reach the bloodstream via the network of blood vessels close to the skin surface which lines the nose. Or the oil can be added to a vaporiser to be breathed in along with air in a room.

Different oils have different effects on the system. For instance, lavender is calming, infection fighting and can also be used as a painkiller and sedative; tea tree is anti-fungal; rose is thought to have a balancing effect on the female hormonal system.

Therapists: To find a professionally qualified therapist in your area contact the Aromatherapy Organisations Council, PO Box 19834, London, SE25 6WF. Tel: 0181 251 7912.

Approx cost: A session costs from £20-45, sometimes more in central London, and will probably last for about 1-1½ hours.

COLOUR THERAPY

Colour therapy is the use of colour to treat physical, mental and emotional problems. It is often combined with other therapies, especially aromatherapy, healing, reflexology and acupuncture, and is based on the fact that each colour vibrates at its own specific frequency, and so do healthy human cells. If an area is diseased or stressed, colour therapists believe that the cells there will vibrate at the wrong frequency rate, but that colour may help restore their healthy cell vibration.

The therapist will choose a colour (from a selection) to help you, the frequency of which is thought to be the same as that of the area which needs restoring and rebalancing. Many therapists also work with the human chakras – the seven major energy centres of the human body. Each chakra has its own specific colour, as well as its own spiritual, emotional and physiological properties – violet for the top of the head; indigo for the forehead; light blue for the throat; green for the heart area etc.

Colour therapists treat people with visualisation and coloured light. Afterwards you are given some homework to do and this is a vital part of the treatment. It usually involves wearing clothes of a particular colour, over a certain area of the body, placing coloured squares of silk next to the skin in certain areas, and visualising colour two or three times a day on the relevant part(s) of your body. Colour therapy has been successfully tested in clinical trials, but not very extensively. Two that demonstrated how it could help people with painful conditions were a study in 1993 which used flashing red lights to head off migraine, with ninety-three per cent of patients saying it did help, and seventy-three per cent reporting that their migraines stopped dead within an hour. Another in 1982 at the San Diego School of Nursing found regular fifteen-minute sessions of blue light produced significant pain relief for middle-aged women suffering from arthritis.

Colour therapists treat people with visualisation and coloured light

Therapists: Colour therapy may not sound that powerful ('Coloured light? Is that all?') but treat it with respect as too much of one colour can adversely affect your health – red especially ought to be used carefully as it can lower your resistance to pain and raise blood pressure. The therapy's governing body proved very elusive when I wrote this book, so your best bet is to contact the Institute of Complementary Medicine on 0171 237 5165 as they have a register of many of the different reputable complementary practitioners in all therapies for the UK.

Approx cost: Sessions cost around £45-50 for sixty to ninety minutes, and approximately £25 for follow-ups.

HERBS

Herbs have been used as medicines for many thousands of years. Some of them are still around as pharmacological medicines – willow bark is a famous anti-inflammatory and has been chemically reproduced as the ubiquitous aspirin; foxglove's active ingredient digitalis is a heart beat regulator and still used in cardiac drugs today.

However scientists' best efforts to separate out and identify every single chemical in medicinal plants (ingredients include the healing agents tannins, bitters and glycosides) have fallen slightly flat because it's not always possible to synthetically reproduce every single one of the components of a herb, and even when possible, it is sometimes at the expense of the original herb's effectiveness and safety.

Supplement and herbal product manufacturers argue that their standardised extracts may in many cases be preferable to 'whole herb or plant use' because plants' levels of active components can vary widely. Some samples have twice the amount of active ingredients than others, some, according to Stephen Terrass, nutritionist and technical director at supplement company Solgar UK, have fifty times the amount, depending on quality. Most traditional herbalists, however, say that it's best to use the natural whole herb rather than manufactured extracts because the whole plant is the medicine and this whole is greater than the sum of its parts. This is why when you take traditional medicinal herbs, it tends to be as a tea made from the entire herb and boiling water, or as a whole-plant tincture or an infusion.

Only about six medical doctors in the UK are also fully trained as herbalists

For those of us who consider a cup of vile-tasting herb tea three times daily to be pretty off-putting, health food and supplement companies also produce the pure powdered herbs in capsule form and as palatable tinctures. These are widely available in health food shops, specialist herbalist shops, and by mail order (see p.144). Different herbs are prescribed for different symptoms – chickweed, marigold or euphrasia for aching sore eyes; black cohosh and cramp bark for period pains; feverfew for migraines. Herbs are also used to keep your entire system generally healthy and balanced. Echinacea (purple cone flower) for instance boosts and backs up the immune system. Many clinical trials have been carried out on herbs as medicines (see p. 146).

Therapists: The National Institute of Medical Herbalists, 56 Longbrooke Street, Exeter EX4 6AH. Tel: 01392 426 022. The training is extensive, but only about six medical doctors in the UK are also fully trained as herbalists, so most will be lay professionals.

Approx cost: Depending on where you live consultations are usually £30-35, but may be as high as £50-60 in central London.

HOMEOPATHY

Homeopathy is based on the principle of 'like cures like'. Though it works gently it can be very powerful and is not only useful for grumbling conditions such as rheumatism but for emergency situations such as accidents, and major events such as childbirth. It is even very safe for small babies.

Minute quantities of a substance which, in a healthy person, would produce the symptoms of the illness you were trying to cure (such as Apis – bee venom – for insect stings and inflamed, hot, itching/burning swellings and rashes) are used as homeopathic medicines. These are thought to work by aggravating the symptoms slightly, which stimulates your body's own get-well defences. And unlike conventional (allopathic) medicine, the lower the dose, the more powerful its effect. Many successful clinical trials have been carried out on the effectiveness of homeopathy (see p. 146). Dosages are described as 'potencies'. The most common and the gentlest is potency six (6c) and remedies are available in major high street chemists, such as Boots. The next one up and very commonly used is 30c, available from homeopathic pharmacies, such as Ainsworths in London and some health shops. A practitioner may give a patient a 200c in an acute situation and these are also available from homeopathic pharmacies by telephone order to members of the public.

Homeopathy is based on the principle of 'like cures like'

The remedies come in the form of white powders, pillules, tiny tablets (most of which is sugar) or tinctures. For the best overall results you should see a well-qualified practitioner, but there are a great many homeopathic remedies you can use at home/decide on yourself, and if it's the wrong remedy it will not harm you, which makes it in many ways an ideal self-help therapy.

Therapists: Homeopathy is available on the NHS in a limited way, but there are also five homeopathic NHS hospitals you can request a referral to: Tunbridge Wells, Glasgow, London, Liverpool and Bristol. For a register of medical doctors trained in homeopathy contact The British Homeopathic Association, 27a Devonshire Street, London W1. Tel: 0171 935 2163. For a lay (non-medical) homeopath contact The Society of Homeopaths, 2 Artizan Road, Northampton NN1 3HR. Tel: 01604 621 400.

Approx costs: Initial consultations lasting from forty-five minutes to one hour usually cost from £30-60, but can reach as high as £120 in London's Harley Street.

NUTRITION/DIET THERAPY

This type of therapy uses diet as a whole (as in an anti-arthritis diet pp. 28-30, or an anti-migraine diet pp. 86-9) or by using individual minerals, vitamins and nutritional supplements to treat illness. The latter is used on the basis that while few people these days in developed countries suffer from full-blown vitamin/mineral deficiencies such as scurvy and rickets, many have slight shortages or sub-clinical deficiencies which can show up as general mild ill health and tiredness, or as aches and pains.

For instance, so far as treating pain with food substances is concerned, glucosamine sulfate can be used for osteo arthritis, and magnesium, vitamin D and calcium for migraines. Both have been subjected to clinical trials. See p. 146 for these and many other references to trials looking at using nutrition to treat pain. Professional therapists may also use a detoxifying programme and allergy/blood/sweat testing, plus a general dietary overhaul rather than just prescribing one or two nutrients in isolation.

The trick is identifying which dietary approach works best for you personally and what your body in particular is lacking. This is where a full medical history, and a careful diagnosis backed up if necessary by the relevant tests carried out by properly qualified therapists or clinical nutritionists, can be invaluable. It's no good spending a hefty sum on what are often expensive nutritional supplements from the best health food shop if you are not taking quite the right supplements or not taking them in the correct quantities for your individual requirements.

You've got two good options for nutritional DIY:

1. See a good nutritional therapist/doctor first and sort out exactly what you need, then get your progress monitored by them.
2. Use your own instincts, knowledge of your body, and background information gathering to see what you feel would be helpful.

Then try it for six weeks or so: you may need to extend this to eight to twelve weeks on some of the special eating plans. If there is no improvement, or you are getting worse, stop taking the tablets and go see a professional. If it's helping, hooray.

Therapists: The Society for the Promotion of Nutritional Therapy, PO Box 85, St Albans, AL3 7ZQ, Tel: 01582 792 088, has a register of professionally trained therapists whose qualifications are accepted by the NHS. Naturopaths are also trained in nutrition: contact the General Council and Register of Naturopaths at Goswell House, 2 Goswell Road, Street, Somerset BA16 0JG. Tel: 01458 840 072.

Approx costs: Anything from £25-100 a session. This excludes fees for any tests.

REFLEXOLOGY

Reflexology is the practice of applying pressure to very specific points on the feet and the hands, to stimulate the body's own healing system. Reflexologists believe that different parts of the body are mirrored on the feet and hands – for instance, the womb area is on the inside of a woman's ankle, the neck area runs down the middle of the underneath of your big toe. There are 70,000 nerve endings on the sole of each foot and when you stimulate these points by touching firmly, rubbing or pressing, a message is sent along the autonomic nerve system's pathways to all areas of the body and brain. The effect of reflexology treatments is cumulative, but you may find that improvements begin following a single session. The therapy has been studied in many clinical trials (see p. 146) on subjects as varied as postal workers with bad backs in Odense (Denmark) in 1993, where sick leave dropped by a quarter; to pain in childbirth, where one piece of London-based research in 1995 showed women receiving reflexology had shorter labours by up to two thirds, and only ten per cent of the usual amount of epidurals.

Reflexologists believe that different parts of the body are mirrored on the feet and hands

According to top reflexologist Farah Begum-Baig who has her own clinic in Cambridge and also teaches doctors and nurses reflexology and stress management at Addenbrookes and Ely NHS Hospital Trusts in Cambridge: 'The ideal way to use reflexology for pain relief is to treat both feet and then to focus on the points corresponding to the specific ailments. It is a truly holistic treatment – it acts on the whole body.

Research in 1995 showed women receiving reflexology had shorter labours by up to two thirds

'The right foot has the reflex points corresponding to the organs on the right side of the body, the left foot has those for the left-hand side of the body. However, just to confuse everyone, "cross reflexes" do exist too. For instance, a tender spot over a reflex point in the right shoulder can refer to the left hip, and there are similar crossovers between the knees and elbows – worth knowing about if someone has tennis elbow pain, or golfer's shoulder.'

Therapists: There are several different regulatory boards, including The British Reflexology Association, Monks Orchard, Whitbourne, Worcester WR6 5RB. Tel: 01886 821 207.

Approx cost: From £15-40 for a forty-five to sixty minute session.

VISUALISATION

This is literally the practice of seeing yourself better in your own mind's eye and concentrating hard on doing so at regular intervals. It's best combined with some relaxation exercises so that your mind is cleared of 'any other business' temporarily leaving it free to concentrate its very considerable power on the matter in hand. Any yoga class or a hypnotherapist or autogenic trainer can teach you how to do this, but if you have no time for anything complicated and time consuming, try the following exercise:

- Lie down or sit comfortably and with your eyes closed and breathe in for a count of eight.
- Hold the breath for eight then breathe out for eight.
- Do this twenty times.
- This exercise is pretty good for getting you in the right frame of mind – relaxed, yet focused.

Systematic relaxation in the form of autogenic training (a form of deep mind/body relaxation), yoga and hypnotherapy has been studied in clinical trials and found to benefit most conditions which have an element of stress influencing them, such as period pain and IBS. It also helps subjects to tolerate pain better (for example, in childbirth, arthritis, and chronic back pain).

Therapists: There is no standard training just in relaxation and visualisation. However, because it is an integrated mind/body discipline, many yoga and meditation classes use and teach gentle, simple techniques as a matter of course. Contact the British Wheel of Yoga, 1 Hamilton Place, Boston Road, Sleaford, Lincs NG34 7ES. Tel: 01529 306 851.

Approx cost: Yoga classes start from £2.50 a session. If you want some more intense and systematic training in visualisation/relaxation from a hypnotherapist or autogenic instructor, see p. 144.

THE A-Z OF COMMON ACHES AND PAINS

ARTHRITIS AND RHEUMATISM

The words 'arthritis' and 'rheumatism' sound as if they are the names of two different, distinct diseases, but they aren't. Both come under the vast umbrella of rheumatic diseases. Arthritis means an 'inflammation of the joints' but the word is often used inaccurately, even when there is no inflammation there at all. Rheumatism is an even more overused term and technically it just describes general aches and pains in muscles/joints.

There are more than 200 types of these rheumatic diseases. They affect one in every thousand children, and hundreds of thousands of young/youngish adults – scuppering the myth that this group of disorders are somehow an unavoidable part of the ageing process. They aren't. Probably the best thing about them is that whether you have the type that lasts a few months or the type that lasts for the rest of your life, there is a great deal that you can do for yourself to help diminish the onset and painful, restricting symptoms by working around many of the limitations they can impose, and sometimes even dampening them down altogether.

For most people, arthritis causes discomfort or pain. The pain varies from the nagging to the exhausting and downright debilitating, and can be referred to an unaffected part of the body or felt at the site of the inflammation itself (for instance some people with arthritis of the hip report that their knee hurts). According to Arthritis Care, there are many different types of 'standard' pain – some people experience it all the time, for others it comes and goes, some feel sharp stabbing pains, others aching or a combination of different aches and pains in different places. Stiffness is another very common symptom. So are tiredness and frustration. Fighting constant pain is exhausting and can leave little energy for much else. Often the frustration at the limitations the condition imposes on your life can be tremendous, reinforced every time you

An integrated approach can combine whatever is needed from orthodox medicine, excercise, nutrition, mind/body medicine and complementary therapies to help you either get better, or to cope far more easily

are unable to twist the top off the coffee jar, have difficulty getting out of a bath or making it up the road to the corner shop.

Because each person reacts differently to pain or to treatment, your particular type of rheumatic disease – whether it's rheumatoid arthritis or gout – its progress, what helps or makes it worse and what effect certain medications may have, will all be very individual. Like other health problems that are more syndromes than single specific disorders (PMS, IBS) what helps depends on what triggered yours personally. There may be several different contributing triggers, which you can track down one by one using a process of inspired deduction, instinct and straight trial/error rather than a single cause. And, as with all multifactorial disorders, it may well benefit from a multifactoral solution. An integrated approach can combine whatever is needed from orthodox medicine, exercise, nutrition, mind/body medicine and complementary therapies to help you to either get better, or to cope extremely well with what you are unable to cure.

DIFFERENT SORTS OF ARTHRITIS

The most common types are:

OSTEOARTHRITIS (OA)

This usually develops gradually over a number of years, affecting several different joints, especially the hands, knees, feet, spine and hips. The cartilage disc in the joint such as the knee thins out, bony outgrowths form on the outer edges of the joint making it look knobbly, the joint becomes progressively stiff, often inflamed as well, and possibly swollen. Treatments include ordinary painkillers and occasionally steroid injections. Eighty per cent of elderly people have some degree of OA.

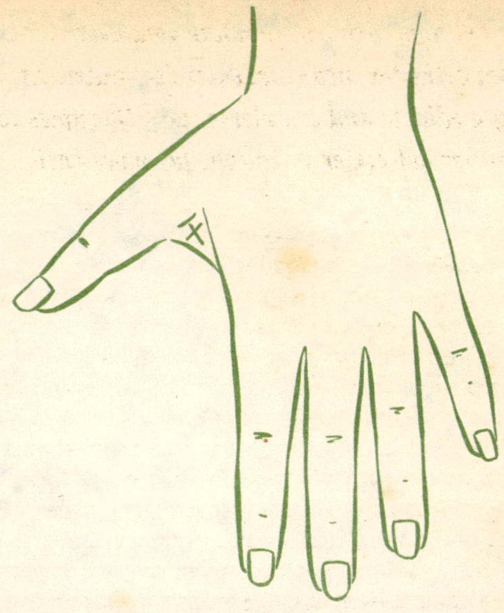

For all-round pain relief locate the Hegu 4 acupressure point as marked. Feel around the fleshy web between your thumb and index finger until you find an especially sensitive spot. Press with the ball of your thumb, rotating gently, for 2–3 minutes at a time, 2–3 times a day. If in a great deal of pain try this every half hour.

SECONDARY ARTHRITIS

This can develop many years after an injury damaged a joint, and is especially common in weight-bearing joints, such as the knee.

RHEUMATOID ARTHRITIS (RA)

This is where the joints become inflamed and painful. Unlike OA, RA people also tend to feel generally tired and unwell, with early-morning stiffness that may last up to several hours. It is thought that it is an auto-immune disease whereby the body's own defence system starts attacking rather than protecting the joints.

RA may build up slowly over several weeks or months, but in a few cases a severe shock or emotional distress can trigger it rapidly, with or without a high fever: some people with RA say that after a particularly stressful time or following an illness, 'I just woke up with it one morning'. It is usually treated with 'disease-modifying anti-rheumatic drugs' (NSAIDs – Non Steroidal Anti-Inflammatory Drugs), sometimes steroids too if things are pretty severe, or with other drugs that suppress the immune system. Anti-malaria drugs, a type of penicillin – and gold – are also used. Ligaments, tendons and muscles may become weak and inflamed, and eventually the joints may become deformed. RA affects two per cent of the population, but women are two to three times as likely to develop it as men.

RA *affects two per cent of the population, but women are two to three times as likely to develop it as men*

GOUT

This is wrongly seen by the unsympathetic as the wages of over indulgence, and the sort of thing which only wealthy old epicures get. Henry VIII had it, and the image of a puce-faced, gouty old monarch with a rib of red beef in one hand and a party-sized flagon of claret in the other has never quite left the national imagination. Gout is caused by uric acid crystals in the joints, not by overeating. Uric acid is a natural waste product and we all have a certain amount of it in our bloodstream, but some people either cannot eliminate it from their systems fast enough or are producing more than is usual. When levels become too high excess uric acid develops into crystals which can form around the joints where they cause inflammation, swelling and often severe pain.

Gout usually attacks the joints at the bottom of the big toe, but it can also affect the ankles, wrists, hands, elbows and knees. It comes on fast. One day the joint in question is aching, the next it can be red, swollen and seriously painful. The bout usually dies away within a week or so. It is treated with anti-inflammatory drugs. Cutting down alcohol and red meat also helps.

ANKYLOSING SPONDYLITIS (AS)

This is another type of inflammatory arthritis, but it begins in the joints of the lower back which become inflamed and stiff. If it is not treated, the spinal joints may fuse together so that you cannot move them at all. The main form of treatment for AS is gentle exercise to relieve the pain and to keep as much flexibility as possible.

YOU CAN MAKE THE DIFFERENCE

None of the orthodox treatments – whether they are painkillers, steroids or gold – will cure arthritis and doctors do not claim they will. What they do (with varying degrees of success) is control the symptoms. It is all the different things that you can do for yourself – such as taking specific nutritional supplements, changing what you eat, relaxation and visualisation – that makes all the extra difference. Self-help therapies can even keep the condition down permanently, and without the (sometimes serious) side effects that the stronger drugs can cause.

WHAT YOU CAN DO FOR YOURSELF

'Prolonged pain has the power to crush our self-confidence and lead us to lose our sense of who we are. It is rather like being trapped in an endlessly revolving door ... *and it may come as a surprise but the only effective way to overcome pain is to do something about it ourselves.*'

Dr Chris Wells, former director of the famous Centre for Pain Relief, at Liverpool's Walton Hospital.

OA AND RA: EAT TO BEAT THEM

DEADLY NIGHTSHADE

Stick to a special eating plan that avoids all the nightshade family: that means no tomatoes, white potatoes, peppers and aubergine. All have a substance called solanine in them which can be toxic if it's not broken down by your intestine. One survey of people with arthritis who avoided eating nightshade foods found that seventy-two per cent of them felt better for it (see p. 146). Though it's never been put to strict clinical tests and can take up to six months to make any difference (if it is going to at all) it remains pretty popular.

ALLERGY SEARCH

Turn detective – might a type of food or food ingredient be setting you off? Although there is more proof for this in the case of RA than OA, it's worth a try if other avenues are turning into dead ends.

THE WARMBRAND WAY

Too strict for some (often the idea is greeted with 'Well what can I eat, then?') but used with some success from the 1950s to '70s, devised by a naturopathic doctor called Max Warmbrand. No meat, eggs or dairy products – now even harder than in Max's heyday – no chemicals, sugar or processed foods. However, the wide range of new soya-based products (burgers, mince, sausages, tofu) and quorn (made from fungi, tastes like chicken) helps balance this, and some are seriously tasty though others taste like seasoned blotting paper. Although there are no clinical trials, there is a bestselling book and reportedly thousands of happy patients.

THINGS TO TAKE FOR IT

If you don't want arthritis in the first place ...

If arthritis seems to run in your family, or if you have an old injury which you suspect may be a starting point for this painful condition later on, such as a damaged knee, taking anti-oxidant vitamins preventatively from now on, especially vitamin C and E, plus the mineral selenium – may help stop you developing the condition at all. They are also said to be a great anti-ageing weapon (looks as well as body systems). Trace elements, such as copper and manganese, may also be important.

THE ARTHRITIS-PREVENTION COCKTAIL

For most people the levels you need in a good anti-arthritis/anti-ageing cocktail are roughly: Vitamin C: 500-2000mg daily; selenium: 100-200 ugs; Vitamin E: 200-400iu; copper: 1-2mg; zinc: 20-25mg; magnesium: 500mg. If that sounds both fiddley and expensive to you (it is) try an all-in-one pill, such as Advanced Antioxidant Formula (Solgar).

KILLING THE PAIN – NATURALLY

None of the following produce the instant result of a powerful painkiller. They are slow but steady builders if they are going to work, but unlike hefty painkillers or steroids, the results can last:

- Think ACE: Yes, it's the anti-oxidant trio again. Offering protection against developing cancer and ageing skin, vitamins A, C and E seem to get everywhere. Vitamin E has specifically been shown to reduce both RA and OA symptoms (see p. 146) and recent research by the Boston University Arthritis Center found that vitamin C could slow down OA too, and that people who ate plenty of vitamin C had three times less chance of getting knee pain than those who didn't.

- Fish oils: These, such as good old-fashioned cod liver oil, contain vital omega three fatty acids, EPA and DHA. Both have a good anti-inflammatory effect, and though more often linked with RA treatment they may also help OA. Watch out for 'fishy burps' though. Capsules are much more palatable, but pricier, than a tablespoon of the stuff – that unmistakable whiff of raw cod has a way of lingering on your tastebuds. Fish oil has the added advantage of being good for your hair and skin too.
- Boron: This mineral is important for helping your body to put any calcium it takes into good bone-building use, and there is a link between being short of boron and developing OA. Research suggests 6mg a day for two months may help.
- The herb boswellia: This is said to be an effective anti-inflammatory but is not linked with gut irritation or ulcers, as prescription NSAIDs are.
- Traditionally, another herb, horsetail, has long been used for arthritis, and so has white willow for its pain relieving effects (do not take this if you are allergic to aspirin).
- An amino acid called D-Phlenylalanine has been used to treat chronic on-going pain (not just from arthritis), mostly using up to 1500 mg daily, but results have been a mixed bag. The side effects can include heartburn or headaches.

BE YOUR OWN HOMEOPATH

For the best results with chronic arthritis you need to see a homeopath, who will probably give you a good constitutional treatment, but for isolated flare-ups the following may help. Take them up to four times daily for a couple of weeks:

Byronia 30c if your pain is severe, if movement and heat make it even worse and cool compresses help.

Aconite 30c is worth trying for nasty flare-ups in cold weather.

Calcarea phos 6c could be useful if your OA joints feel chilly and numb, and your stiffness is worse when the weather changes.

Rhus tox 6c could be the one for you if heat helps but cold and damp makes it all worse, and if the pain wears off when you move about but the stiffness is worse in the morning.

OA ONLY

- ***Glucosamine sulfate*:** This is a nutrient made from sea shells and contains the building blocks that are needed for repairing joint cartilage. Studies (see p. 146-7) suggest OA symptoms lessen and damaged joints start being repaired if people take 500mg three times daily, but don't expect to see results for three to eight weeks. The situation deteriorates again if you stop taking it.
- ***Cartilage supplement, green lipped mussel and chondroitin sulfate* (CS):** Anyone who has high blood pressure, any form of heart disease or circulation problems should not take CS, which makes it unsuitable for many older people as these disorders can all become increasingly common with age.
- ***Colour therapy*:** Try orange over the areas that are affected: colour therapists say that it is both warming and that it may help to calm some of the inflammation. Interestingly, orange/yellow metals and spices have also been shown to reduce inflammation and to help arthritis and rheumatism – see gold, copper and turmeric, p. 30-31. So if it's the knees that are affected: try cotton orange tights; if it's the feet and ankles: orange socks, if it's in the hips: again orange tights or an orange silk top or underfoot (dyed), which covers them beneath your clothes. This is not so for RA sufferers if the joints are very inflamed – they are quite warm enough already and the orange just may make things a bit worse.

Try orange over the areas that are affected

Smart Eating:
The red-light foods to avoid or considerably cut back on if you have OA include: fried foods, dairy products (go for very low fat or fat free if you can) tomatoes, booze, tobacco, caffeine, spuds, aubergines, peppers (black pepper is OK), refined white sugar, and red meats, such as beef and lamb.

RA ONLY

HERBAL CUPPAS

Try drinking herbs such as devil's claw and burdock root. Devil's claw has not been researched especially scientifically – none of those double blind, placebo-controlled trials which doctors and discerning consumers understandably like to see backing up a treatment – but it has traditionally been used as a treatment for RA for many hundreds of years, possibly because it seems to have an anti-inflammatory effect. Do not take it if you are pregnant.

Diuretic drinks, such as celery seed tea, can also help eliminate toxins and excess fluid which may collect around the joints, causing pressure build up and yet more discomfort

Burdock was, in the old days, thought to help clear the bloodstream of toxins. Traditional herbalists suggest 2-4ml of burdock root tincture a day, and if the dried root is in capsule form, it's usually taken as 1-2g three times a day. Commonly suggested amounts of Devil's Claw are 500-1000 mg twice daily. Diuretic drinks, such as celery seed tea, can also help eliminate toxins and excess fluid which may collect around the joints, causing pressure build up and yet more discomfort.

> To make celery seed tea: Bring to the boil 1oz celery seeds in two pints of water and simmer for twenty minutes. Strain and drink one small cup three times daily.

- **A *low-fat eating plan*:** Certain types of fat (such as animal fats) can trigger an auto-immune reaction and inflammation, and some types can inhibit it. As RA is an auto-immune disease, a diet that is as low as taste permits in animal fat can help. Some people have also found that low-fat, pure vegetarian diets did the trick for them (see p. 147), others found that avoiding gluten (anything made of wheat, rye, oats or barley) made a real difference. Talk to a good nutritionist about devising an eating plan for you which is as tasty and practical to follow as possible, because really hard-to-follow boring diets tend to get broken after the first few weeks.

- ***Turmeric and ginger*:** Find that a veggie diet helps, but feel it's bland? Spice it up with turmeric (the yellow/orange spice that is used in brightly coloured curry dishes), as it is known to protect the body from free radicals, and to have an anti-inflammatory effect. Ginger may also be a good additive – it's much used in Indian Ayurvedic medicine as an anti-inflammatory.
- ***Evening primrose oil, or starflower (borage) oil*:** These oils may help as they contain a substance called GLA (gamma lineolic acid) a known anti-inflammatory. Some double-blind research trials (in which no one knew what they were taking, or even if they were taking an active ingredient or the dummy medication) showed combining evening primrose oil with fish oil works well too.
- ***Yucca*:** Yes, those stoic-looking desert plants usually owned by people who never remember to water them. Fortunately for yuccas, they are even harder to kill than the ubiquitous spider plant. They are related to the Joshua Tree and Native American Indians made poultices out of yucca for all sorts of inflammation, including RA. The usual dosage for modern tablets or capsules is 1000-1500mg daily, unless you want to go to the trouble of boiling up a quarter oz of the roots in a pint of water for fifteen minutes, and drink three to five cups a day – which you probably don't.

SMART EATING FOR RA

Avoid or cut right back on:

Fried foods, dairy foods unless they are very low fat or fat free, tobacco, caffeine (that's tea, coffee and colas) spuds, any foods you seem to feel worse for eating as you may be allergic to them, red meats, tomatoes, aubergines and peppers. Black pepper as a seasoning is fine.

GOLD AND COPPER

Warming yellow and orange metals gold and copper can help, whether it's a copper bangle on your wrist or a gold ring on your finger and sceptics note – it's not just folklore – clinical trials and reports have backed this up (see p. 147). Copper acts as an anti-inflammatory agent as it's needed to kick-start an enzyme called superoxide dismutase (SOD), whose job it is to protect the joints from inflammation. People with RA are often short of copper in their bodies. And gold? Keep that wedding ring on – better still, wear one on each digit, such as some traditional rich Indian and Arabic women do at parties. Research by the City Hospital in Birmingham suggests the gold could pass through the skin 'downstream' to the nearest knuckle joint in big enough quantities to delay arthritis in that area. Gold has also been used to treat rheumatic diseases since the beginning of this century and is now given both by mouth and injection. Gold salt injections help around sixty per cent of people with RA but one third of all patients do develop severe side effects.

Warming yellow and orange metals gold and copper can help, whether it's a copper bangle on your wrist or a gold ring on your finger

WHAT YOU CAN DO

AROMATHERAPY

Medical aromatherapist Dr Vivienne Lunny recommends mixing two drops each of ginger (for its warming effect), juniper (to encourage the removal of toxins) and rosemary (to encourage good blood circulation) in a palmful of carrier oil and rubbing the mixture on the areas that hurt. It is also good for a back massage.

ACUPRESSURE

Painful knees?

There is a special acupressure spot you can use yourself to help soothe knee joint pain and arthritis of the knee. The Chinese call it Yanglingquan, or Gall Bladder meridian 34. It sits an inch or so below your knee on the outer side of your leg. Feel around that spot with your fingertip until you find the most sensitive point, and use your thumb or fingertip to work on it in small rotating movements for four minutes. Have a twenty minute break then do this again. Repeat as necessary, but it should begin to help after twenty to thirty minutes.

The arthritis 'special'

To help generate your body's own natural painkilling substances, find the special Qiuxu (or GB 40) point on the outside of your ankle. Feel around there until you find the most sensitive spot, and then work it gently but firmly by rotating the ball of your thumb over it for about four minutes. Take a twenty minute break. Repeat as necessary.

The prince of painkillers

If you are feeling too stiff and sore to bend down and scrabble around your ankle for the GB 40, try the easy-access prince of painkillers Hegu 4. This point is used almost more than any other acupressure point on the entire body and helps generate general all-round pain relief (it's like taking a painkilling drug). It lies snuggled between the index and first finger, on the fleshy web between them.

AND FINALLY...THINGS TO SMOKE FOR IT

Cannabis, marijuana, dope, hash...call it what you like, this seems to help many with chronic pain when all else has failed. Medical trials on its use for tooth extraction, root canal work, cancer, and heat injury have confirmed it can work well as a painkiller (see p. 148) but there seems to have been no major research specifically on arthritis and cannabis. However, as there are a good many anecdotal reports of the substance being used successfully to control arthritis pain, the possibility of cannabis as a medicine may be of interest to people with certain types of rheumatic disease who are not being helped sufficiently by ordinary prescription drugs, or who are worried about the side effects of the high dosages they are needing to take long term.

Illegal it may be, but many UK doctors are now aware that cannabis can be useful for a wide variety of conditions not only as a painkiller, but as an anti-sickness agent (for people undergoing certain types of cancer therapy) and an anti-spasticity agent for certain types of neurological disease such as Parkinson's. They are so well aware of it that even The British Medical Association – an organisation not noted for its radicalism – has recently voted in favour of doctors being permitted to prescribe it if the present law was changed, which meant that they could prescribe it for their patients without facing prosecution. In 1991, an anonymous survey of the very respectable American Society of Clinical Oncology also found half of them backing its prescription, and having suggested to patients on the quiet that they try it.

HOW TO GET IT?

As with a really good specialist doctor or dentist, it is informed personal recommendation that really helps. If you are not a regular, or occasional, cannabis smoker, ask anyone who might be: your friends, or your teenage or twenty- and thirty-something children/grandchildren (if you have any). Or try visiting a head shop (a specialist shop selling accessories for smoking cannabis such as papers and pipes, plus books and magazines, which many major cities have). One of the pressure groups for the legalisation of cannabis (see p. 143) may be able to suggest one in your area.

When you get there, perhaps try initially showing an interest in the magazines they stock as a tactful opener, then express your disappointment that the companies advertising in the small ads at the back of these publications only supply seeds, which you would have to cultivate your own supply from, rather than resin or herb thereby having to wait many months for (variable) results. Explain your situation – that you are in chronic pain, that orthodox drugs only help in a limited way and that after hearing some positive anecdotal reports you would like to try a natural alternative – in a quiet moment to the shop assistant, as the shops are usually small and the staff, friendly enthusiasts. They may well be able to advise you further.

WHAT DO YOU DO WITH IT?

As with any drug, different people react in different ways to it, and it may or may not suit you. Also, some batches may have a different effect to others as they are not produced/grown in a controlled, uniform way, as orthodox medicinal drugs are. Anecdotal reports (I also have some advice from two highly respectable, older relatives who currently use it for their chronic, painful osteo- and rheumatoid arthritis) suggest that if you make a herbal tea from it as Queen Victoria used to for her period pains you need the dried herb form (grass or weed) in the strongest variety available. History has not recorded what Victoria's doctor called it, but right now top of the range cannabis in dried leaf form is known as skunk or super skunk.

As to dosage, people tend to work out the appropriate dosage by body weight. For instance, an eight-stone woman might perhaps begin with half a teaspoon in a teacup of boiling water, let it steep for ten minutes, strain and drink slowly before going to bed. If this has no soothing effect upon the pain, the next night, try three-quarters of a teaspoon. An average sized twelve- to thirteen-stone man would probably need nearer a whole teaspoon. If it makes you feel at all unwell, do not try any more.

If you are smoking the cannabis instead you would need to do so either in a small pipe, neat or with tobacco; or in a hand-rolled cigarette, mixed with either the mildest tobacco you can find (split open a Silk Cut Extra Mild) or better still, to avoid the use of nicotine altogether, use a small amount of neat cannabis herb. If this makes too strong a smoke, try a herbal tobacco substitute from the health shop. Tobacco is also a member of the nightshade family – another good reason for trying to avoid it (see p. 25).

The smoking method means that the herb travels directly from the alvioli air sacs of your lungs to your bloodstream, so reaching your system faster than the tea form, so the effects are felt within one to twenty minutes rather than thirty minutes to an hour. Start with only a very little, to work out how much is needed to have an effect on you personally. Do not smoke the entire herbal cigarette at once. Just try a few deep puffs, taking the smoke well down into your lungs, then wait for half an hour or so and see how you feel, as the side effects of cannabis can include disorientation, anxiety and visual disturbance. One or two clinical trials have also reported it can also make someone's perception of pain even sharper. After waiting, if you then feel you need some more, try it.

If you prefer to smoke the cannabis rather than to make a herbal tea from it, you could use it either in its herbal or resin form (which known as hash or dope.). Scrape off a little, enough to sprinkle over most of the tobacco substitute or ultra mild real tobacco in the hand-rolled cigarette. The strength and effect of different resins vary, so again, experiment with a very little and work gently upwards if necessary. The fiddly process of making a marijuana cigarette may be out of the question if the arthritis has affected your hands. However, its one advantage is that resin is easier to find, and cheaper than good-quality skunk. Broad-minded medical specialists suggest that people with breathing problems such as emphysema, bronchitis, asthma etc. should try the tea rather than smoke anything in case this aggravates their respiratory condition. You can also, as with any herb or spice, cook with marijuana, making anything from mince (fry it up gently in the fat from the meat as it first cooks) to rock cakes or fudge, but again the effect can be very variable, the dose may be too high and the result may be too powerful for comfort.

The side effects of cannabis can include disorientation, anxiety and visual disturbance

It may seem that for a small book with very limited space available there is a lot of space devoted to this subject. That is because this particular sort of information can be difficult to come by elsewhere in the normal run of things. It is also because this option is one which appears to have helped many – and for anyone seriously considering trying cannabis as a painkiller it's necessary to have the 'where' and 'how' as well as the 'what to do with it'.

BACK PAIN

Back pain or neck pain are probably the most common health problems there are, along with a headache and a temperature. Many attacks arrive suddenly and sharply, but one in every three adults – and children – becomes a chronic (long-term) back pain casualty. And the fact that this costs industry £5 billion in lost production every year is nothing to the amount of distress and loss in quality of life constant back pain can bring to either the person themselves, or to their family. The bad thing about backache is that it can be hard to treat if it becomes chronic, but the good news is that there are many effective pain calming options for back pain, which you can do for yourself.

Symptoms vary but they may include a dull, deep ache, a vicious stabbing sensation, muscle spasms, shooting pains down the legs and if your lower back is affected your shoulders will often knot and harden painfully in sympathy. Backache usually strikes because a muscle or muscle group in your back has over strained or been injured in some way. The list of potential culprits is long, and includes a vertebrae out of alignment with its fellows in the spine, a pulled ligament, a damaged or misplaced disc, or muscle tension which, if it goes on long enough, irritates and inflames the nerves running through it by clamping tightly around them.

Back pain costs industry £5 billion in lost production every year

Common causes include pregnancy, childbirth, poor working position, poor muscle tone – especially the abdominals as these act almost like guy ropes to keep the back in place – stress/depression which may make the back muscles tense up, and being very overweight. Osteoporosis, hairline fractures, lumbago (pain in the mid-back just below the waist) sciatica (which radiates from lower back to buttock, then down the leg) and arthritis are also common causes.

MOBILE PHONES ARE A PAIN IN THE NECK

You probably know to your cost that hands-free phone calls, clamping your phone between cheek and shoulder while your hands are busy elsewhere, gives you neckache and upper back/shoulder spasm. But it can be a lot more serious than that. One Parisian woman found to her horror that after a thirty-two minute conversation with her cordless phone positioned just so while ironing, she had blocked off her own carotid artery.

SELF-HELP FOR ACUTE ATTACKS:

IF YOUR BACK HURTS DO:

- Pay attention to the pain. It's trying to tell you something important – probably to stop what you are doing. For instance, if you are just finishing off a complicated piece of word processing, do not be tempted to do just another half an hour if your back is beginning to hurt. If you're gardening, don't give it another quarter of an hour to make the most of the dying light. Get up, stretch gently and lie down for a bit, or at least ease yourself into a more comfortable position.

Frozen peas or sweetcorn make a great ice-pack – bash out any lumps first

COMFORTABLE WAYS TO LIE DOWN: Immediately the pain hits try lying face down on the floor, knees bent, with your hands at your sides. This takes the pressure off your back, the force of which is at its greatest sitting, then standing – then lying. If this is not comfortable, try lying on your side with a pillow between your knees, and perhaps another one supporting your lower back or abdomen – especially good if you are several months pregnant. Or try lying on your back with a flattish pillow under your neck and your knees slightly bent, supported, if it feels more comfortable, with a soft cushion.

- Make a rapid DIY ice pack with some frozen sweetcorn or peas with the lumps bashed out, and a thin tea-towel wrapped around it. Put the pack on the part that hurts, but not for more than ten minutes at a time. After ten minutes try applying gentle warmth, from a covered hot water bottle. Some people find just the ice pack helps, others just the heat, others that alternating the two works best for them.
- Go to bed if humanly possible, for a day or two, to give the back as much rest as you can. If you are still flat out after two days, call your GP. You need to have a firm mattress, or to have someone put a mattress on the floor for you. Do not, whatever you do, lie on a waterbed.
- Take the recommended amounts of pain killers at the regular intervals though not more often than the packet advises (even when you wake during the night to keep the levels of painkilling agents in your system topped up).
- If there are no painkillers available and you cannot get out to buy any, have one strong alcoholic drink and lie down, or if comfortable, get into a warm bath. This may be especially helpful if a muscle or muscle group has gone into spasm, as alcohol is initially a muscle relaxant and so is heat. Do not overdo the booze, however: it also acts as an anaesthetic and you do not want to get up and start moving about, only to really damage your

back with an ill-judged movement. 'Feeling no pain' means what it says – in the old days before anaesthetics, a skinful was used during surgery for limb amputations, and as a painkiller in childbirth. (The latter was often disastrous as alcohol crosses the placenta, and tended to suppress the new baby's breathing.)

IF YOUR BACK HURTS DO NOT:

- Carry on regardless
- Be too brave
- Try to work/run/garden through the pain. It is not going to go away on its own
- Ignore your back pain. If it's been there, constantly, for several days on end, see your doctor.

COMFORT POSITIONS FOR ACHING BACKS

Been sitting badly all day? Aching, griping back? Don't just flop down on the sofa in front of the TV to relax, that's just giving your poor back more of the same. Try the Hatha-yoga based Cat Stretch. Get down on all fours, and slowly arch and relax your back. Pregnant and your back's complaining? Lie down with a cushion under your head and your legs up over a chair at right angles.

NATURAL PAIN BUSTERS:

Seventy per cent of people who turn to painkillers still suffer terrible pain, according to Dr Chris Wells, former director of the pioneering Centre for Pain Relief, at Liverpool's Walton Hospital. So if the usual approaches aren't working – why not consider some alternative forms of pain relief?

WHEN THE DRUGS DON'T WORK...

- ***White willow complex*:** This is similar to aspirin but longer lasting and less irritating to the gut.
- **TENS *machines*:** This is a mild electrical stimulation of the body's own powerful natural painkilling substances, using a machine the size of a Walkman. Try renting or borrowing one before you splash out on actually buying a machine, as some people find them very helpful, others, not at all (see p. 145 for a company which will let you have a free three-week trial).
- **DIY *reflexology*:** See the diagram for the area of the foot which

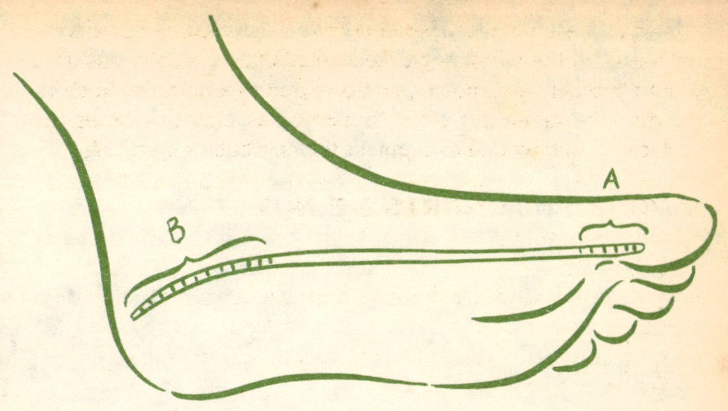

For neck pain relief using reflexology. Press along area A gently but firmly with your *index* finger for 3 minutes, 5 times a day. To help calm lower-back pain (lumbar region). Press and stroke firmly with your thumb along area B for 3 minutes, 5 times a day.

corresponds to the spine – the area to work for lower backache is nearer the ankle, the area for shoulder pain and neckache is towards the big toe.

- **D-*Phenylalanine* (DPA):** Research with chronic pain patients who were taken off all their usual medications found their pain cut by fifty per cent. Watch out for edgy side effects though, which include the jitters, anxiety, headaches (taken on empty stomach) and higher blood pressure (taken with food). It takes two to twenty-one days to see a result – if you are going to – taking 250mg half an hour before your meals, three times daily. If you are having acupuncture for back pain, DPA is an option especially well worth trying as it enhances the effect of the needles.
- **L-*Tryptophan*:** This may be helpful if you have a milder, nagging, persistent pain, but not for anything thunderous. Try 1-4g daily for a month, taken with a simple carbohydrate fruit juice (avoid eating any form of protein for an hour and a half afterwards). If you are also needing to take morphine-based drugs, however, it may stop them being so helpful. This product has not been available in the UK over the counter since 1990 (some Japanese-manufactured products were contaminated and caused

If you are having acupuncture for back pain, DPA *is an option especially well worth trying as it enhances the effect of the needles*

problems worldwide) but is apparently due to be back on the market soon.

- ***Selenium and vitamin* E:** Backache? You may be short on the trace element selenium. Vitamin E, for some reason, helps too, according to one piece of research carried out in 1985 on eighty-one people who had put up with 'disabling muscular pain, stiffness and aching of long duration'. The dosage used is usually about 200ug (*not* mg) of selenium and approx 100mg vitamin E daily.
- ***Yoga*:** Think about taking up gentle yoga to improve your strength and flexibility.
- ***See a good chiropractor or osteopath*:** These are not therapies you can do for yourself but you can self refer to a practitioner.
- ***Exercise*:** Try and take gentle regular exercise. Swimming is great, even if it's only a very little at a time, as your body is also supported by the water's natural buoyancy.
- ***Relaxation*:** Try to do a deep relaxation period daily or if possible, twice daily. A yoga teacher could suggest some very simple techniques as they all use them in standard yoga classes. More structured, deep relaxation such as Autogenic Training or Transcendental Meditation (TM) could help greatly. Whatever you do, regular practice is vital. It's not how much, it's how often.

THERAPEUTIC CANNABIS FOR CHRONIC, INTRACTABLE PAIN

Think about trying cannabis either in a tisane tea form, or smoked (see p. 32-5). Anecdotally it is currently used by people with severe back pain, MS spasticity, cancer-related pain and certain types of painful neurological disease.

GINGER AND JAM

Some research suggests ginger can help the joint inflammation which is the curse of many a bad back. According to work by Odense University, you need half a gram of powdered ginger three times daily (it's available in capsule form from health shops) – or if you are really keen, five whole grams of fresh peeled ginger daily can be helpful. The researchers put it in jam on morning toast, in milk or in natural yoghurt, and apparently it tasted great.

> *Some research suggests ginger can help the joint inflammation which is the curse of many a bad back*

LONG-TERM HELP FOR CHRONIC PAIN

Ask your GP to refer you to one of the specialist pain units in the country for expert help and management/support programmes which integrate orthodox medicine (painkilling drugs, physiotherapy, gentle exercise such as swimming, even surgery) with complementary medicine (acupuncture, osteopathy and chiropractic being some of the most effective for back pain). At these pain units you can also, if you would like to, learn about ways to manage and take control of your back pain, your own way. If you do not feel you need to go to a pain unit but would like to see a trained clinician who specialises in back health, see a good osteopath or chiropractor to discover if it is a structural alignment problem, which they can help with. If it is, you can sometimes feel some improvement right away, even after a single treatment.

BREAST PAIN AND BREAST-FEEDING DISCOMFORT

ORDINARY BREAST PAIN

Half of all women go to their doctors at some point because their breasts are hurting. The most usual problem is cyclical mastalgia – the pain that may arrive in the second half of your menstrual cycle as your breasts gradually become fuller, more sensitive to the touch and also perhaps temporarily lumpier. The second most common problem is the bosom lumpiness that some women find they have all the time, no matter what stage of their menstrual cycle they are in, and which doctors call fibrocystic breast disease.

The first has no link whatsoever with breast cancer, the second, only rarely. However, it's best always to have any persistent lumpiness checked out promptly by your doctor.

WHAT HELPS?

Avoid caffeine

The bad news for all cappuccino addicts is that it really helps to stop drinking caffeine – that's all tea, chocolate, colas, even decaffeinated coffee – and proper coffee most of all. Go for herb teas (rosehip tea bags are one of the strongest and most palatable). Appalled coffee lovers, don't ignore this one – it's helped a lot of women (see p. 148). If you can't wake up without a large mug of caffeine, try a different mental wake-up strategy: perhaps a cool (not cold) face and neck splash and a sniff of geranium, then lemongrass essential oil straight from the bottle.

Cool lavender compresses

When the swelling is at its worst, add ten drops of lavender essential oil to a small basin of cool water, soak a clean flannel in it and apply to your breasts. Lavender has an anti-inflammatory and a pain-killing effect.

Take essential fatty acids

Try evening primrose oil (EPO) or starflower oil: 500-1,000mg three times daily, either all month or just the ten days before your period begins. As this can work out to be expensive, it's worth knowing your GP can prescribe this for you (as 'Efamast') as long as it's for breast pain, not general PMS, which EPO also helps. Watch out for possible mild diarrhoea at high doses.

Healing bras!

Colour therapists suggest wearing green- or turquoise-coloured bras (soothing/cooling) or wearing squares of silk in these colours tucked around the breast inside your bra. Lingerie experts recommend a supportive, comfy bra without underwiring – this is no time for a Wonderbra or a balconette – and getting fitted by an expert fitter (e.g. at a John Lewis', or a specialist underwear shop.) According to a major survey by lingerie manufacturers, eight out of ten women are currently in the wrong bra size, which is likely to make sore breasts even more uncomfortable.

Try lavender essential oil flannel compresses

Eat food that's high in complex carbohydrates, high fibre and low fat

That's lots of fruit, raw vegetable, wholemeal pastas, breads, and brown rice. Try Quorn, tofu and fish instead of red meat, and go for low-fat dairy products only – reduced-fat Greek yoghurt, cottage cheese and skimmed milk. If you are really in pain, try cutting out dairy completely for two months then slowly reintroduce them one by one and see if this makes a difference.

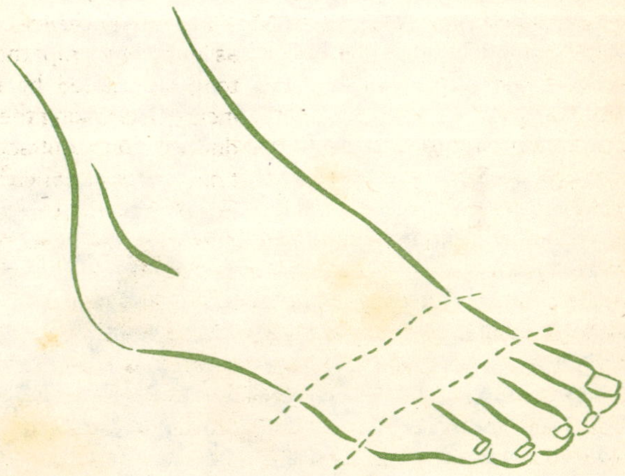

To relieve breast pain using reflexology. Press and smooth your thumb firmly down on this area for 3 minutes at a time, every hour. For added effect you could also work gently on the area corresponding to your womb area (see diagram for period pain relief, pg 111).

***Take extra vitamin* A *and* E**

Several studies report that an additional 200-600iu of vitamin E a day can help. If it's going to make a difference it should have begun to do so after three months.

Colour therapists suggest wearing green- or turquoise-coloured bras (soothing/cooling)

Castor oil packs

Granny's traditional (and vile-tasting) remedy for an upset stomach makes a great breast pack, says holistic obstetrician and gynaecologist Dr Christine Northrup of the pioneering Woman to Woman clinic in Yarmouth, Maine USA. Applying the pack three times a week for an hour over two to three months can often eliminate the problem entirely; thereafter keep up a maintenance level of once a week.

A castor oil (also known as Palma Christi, or the Palm of Christ) pack is made by soaking a flannel in castor oil, placing the saturated flannel directly onto the skin. Cover it with a piece of plastic eg. a plastic bag; then put a hot water bottle or heat pad on top. Wrap the entire area in a towel to keep everything in place. Apply three times a week for one hour over a period of two to three months, suggests Dr Northrup.

If you are really in pain, try cutting out dairy completely for two months

Homeopathy

The following remedies may help – take every twelve hours for up to seven days:

N*atrum mur.* 30 if breasts hurt because they are full and large due to fluid retention.

C*onium.*30 if breasts are large, and both painful and tender.

C*arbo an.* 30 *c* if breasts are large, with shooting pains.

HOW TO TACKLE PREMENSTRUAL PUFFINESS

This contributes to swollen breasts, and swollen breasts tends to mean sore breasts. If you can reduce general water retention you will, as an added plus, no longer have premenstrual doughnut-shaped knees.

- Cut down on salty foods. This reduces water retention in all areas, especially fatty areas such as the breasts.

- Take a vitamin B6 supplement (check the new guidelines on this one).
- As a mild diuretic drink a DIY herbal tea made from one teaspoon of the herb cleavers, steeped for three minutes in a cup of boiling water (see mail-order stockists p. 144)

THE SELLOTAPE AND CABBAGE CURE

Take two leaves of a Savoy cabbage (ordinary green cabbage is no help at all) wash and roll it out hard with a rolling pin. Tuck one into each side of your bra, covering as much of your breast as possible – luckily they are curved so tend to fit pretty well. Or, lightly crush some fresh comfrey leaves the same way, fold them into two light cotton cloths (a man's cotton hankie is perfect for this), dampen lightly and Sellotape them around each breast inside your bra. Leave for an hour. These methods are said to be extremely soothing.

BREAST-FEEDING SORENESS

For newly breast-feeding mothers:

TACKLING SORENESS AND PAIN DUE TO ENGORGEMENT AS THE MILK COMES IN FOR THE FIRST TIME:

- Try alternating hot and cold flannels. Optional: Add ten drops of lavender essential oil to the hot water and cold water in which you soak the flannels.
- Sitting in a warm bath with your breasts under water.
- Smoothing on vitamin E oil very gently to help soothe the stretching feeling.
- Savoy cabbage leaves (above). Wear over your breasts or tucked underneath your bra (Egyptian midwives actually did a trial on this in 1987).
- Cucumber slices contain anti-inflammatory, cooling agents which is why they are also useful for sunburn. Rumour has it that TV chat show host Vanessa Feltz swears by sliced strawberries too. However, they can stain, squash and/or make you feel like you have a maternity bra full of fruit salad – especially if you also have the cucumber slices down there.

SORE BREAST-FEEDING NIPPLES?

- Dry your nipples* after each feed very gently by either shining a high wattage bulb heat on them (anglepoise lamps are best for this) or dabbing (not rubbing) them gently with cotton wool.
- Anoint with calendula cream (like Kamilosan) after each feed. Calendula soothes soreness and speeds healing, thus helping to prevent the problem from recurring.
- The same (above) applies to petroleum gel, like Vaseline.
- Keep your nipples as dry as possible – change nipple pads very often – carry a supply in your handbag/jeans pocket.
- When practical, open your nursing bra cups, keeping the bra's structural support in place, and let the air circulate.
- Ask your local midwife or breast-feeding counsellor (NCT, La Leche) to come and check if your baby is latching on to you in the right position when feeding – this can make all the difference between nipples that feel like they've had hot peppers rubbed into them and complete comfort.
- Homeopathy – the following may be of help:
  Chamomilla 6c for inflamed/tender nipples.
  Sulphur 6c for cracked nipples that are really smarting.
  Graphites 6c for cracked and blistered nipples. (1 pillule to be taken every four hours for up to six doses, suggests homeopathic GP and author Dr Andrew Lockie.)
- Mix ten drops of lavender essential oil into a palmful of bland carrier oil (soya oil will do) and smooth onto your breasts. Lavender is soothing, mildly analgesic and helps to prevent and treat infection.

*NIPPLES AND HAIRDRYERS

Warning: if a friend recommends you blast them with a hairdryer on a low setting (once considered good alternative advice), think twice. Sore nipples have tiny cracks, and germs can find their way in through these easily, causing infection and more soreness. A hairdryer's moving parts may not be the most sterile of objects, so the air blown over your nipples could cause infection.

NIPPLE NOTES

Infection, such as candida (yes, thrush – it gets everywhere) can cause extreme nipple soreness for breast-feeding mothers. Suspect

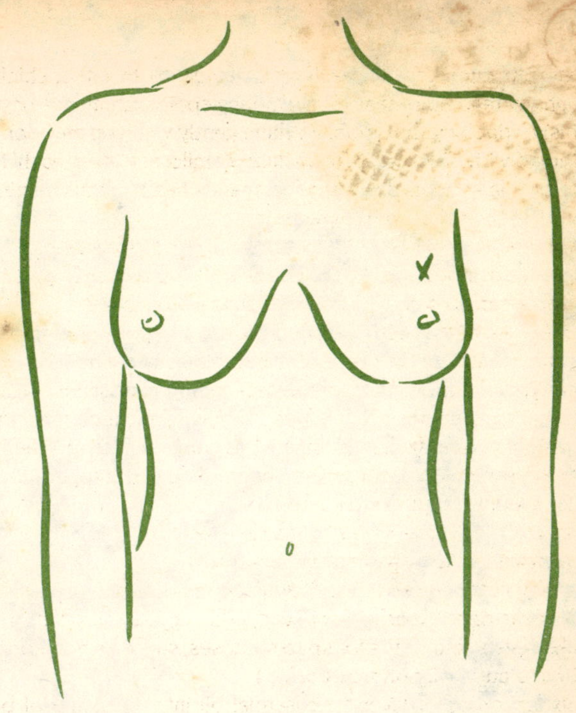

For helping calm breast and chest pain, and for breastfeeding problems such as mastitis. Press the area at the top of your breast, in line with your nipple, as marked. Apply gentle pressure for between 30 seconds and 2 minutes, using your middle or index finger. (It may be easier to slide your thumb under your armpits for support.)

nipple thrush if they are not healing no matter how dry and Vaselined you keep them; and if the sore red area is beginning to extend past your areola (the coloured part of the nipple) or if the nipples appear very red. Check with your GP. If it is nipple thrush it needs anti-candida cream treatment. Or you can get the same Canesten anti-fungal cream your GP would probably give you from the pharmacist without prescription.

POWDER YOUR NIPPLES?

The natural DIY approach is to lightly cover the nipples with lactobacillus acidophilus powder, available in freeze-dried capsule format (see pp. 144-5) plus cooled natural, live yoghurt and do the same for your baby's mouth, checking for any tell-tale curdy white discharge at the corners, or redness and soreness. Gently wash and dry your nipples after each feed, then smooth on the powder and yoghurt.

THRUSH BOTTOM RECIPE FOR BABIES

Intractable nappy rash with redness and itching, plus a tiny sprinkling of pink pinhead spots around the solid red rash area may be thrush infection. Try the yoghurt and acidophilus recipe (above) as this can help balance out any excess growth of candida. If possible leave the baby's nappy off for as long as is practical each day providing your home/the weather are warm enough. If the condition hasn't improved markedly in three days, it's best to go and check with your GP.

BUNIONS

Unglamorous they may be, but a spot of bunion trouble is a fact of life for anyone who's spent the last twenty years flaunting fashionable shoes, unless their choice was a pair of differently coloured twelve-hole Doc Martins for every occasion. A bunion is a lay term for what doctors call hallux valgus, which is basically the protrusion of the first big toe joint at an angle. Over that joint is a fluid-filled sac or bursa, which usually gives the joint some protection against friction. Too much friction though, and it becomes inflamed and painful.

The problem is that when feet are crammed into shoes which look great but simply aren't feet-shaped around the toes (i.e. they

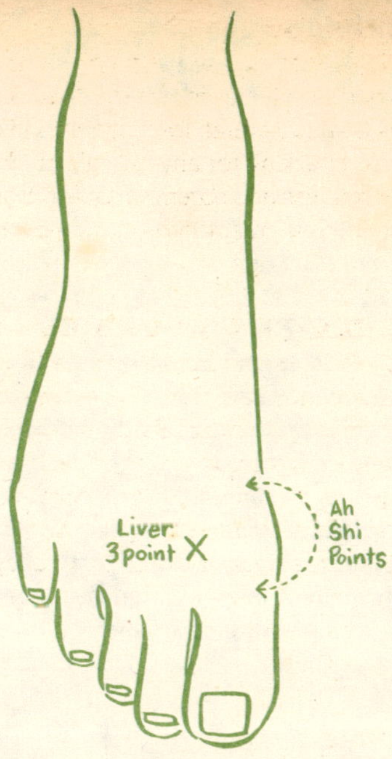

Help soothe bunion pain by gently pressing what Chinese acupuncturists call the Ah Shi point for 2-3 minutes at a time, 3 times a day. These are local, tender areas. Also, gently work the Liver 3 point for the same amount of time.

narrow sharply to make the foot look sexy and dainty) this pushes the toes in to fit the space available, and the first big toe joint is left compressed at an angle on the outside of the foot. Fashion shoes often have high heels too, which tip your entire body weight down on to your toes, increasing pro-bunion pressure.

As the protruding joint pushes against the shoe, hard skin grows over it to form a callus, and the longer this type of shoe is worn, the more firmly the new angle of the foot becomes fixed – it literally has no choice but to grow to fit. Eventually prolonged shoe pressure makes the bursa fill with fluid, which can become painfully inflamed or infected (a condition known as bursitis). Suddenly the only things that are really comfortable to wear are trainers.

Dissolve a tablespoon of Epsom salts in a bowl of hot water, and soak your feet in it

TAKING THE B****! OUT OF BUNIONS

- To help ease joint soreness dissolve a tablespoon of Epsom salts in a bowl of hot water, and soak your feet in it.
- Massage the area gently after soaking.
- If it's swollen, apply cold compresses three times daily. Cold compresses can help take the heat out of any swelling – try distilled witch-hazel (from the chemist), or one made with a single drop of homeopathic arnica tincture in a little water. The quickest way to make a compress is to soak a clean flannel in the healing liquid you have prepared, and apply.
- Massage on comfrey or arnica cream.
- Make your own soothing poultice with up to 1 tbsp dried or fresh comfrey herb, and use to calm the area and reduce swelling. Chop up the herb finely (or put in a blender). Add a little boiling water and mix to a paste. Put in between two pieces of gauze, and bind it around your bunion and foot with a cotton bandage. Tip: this method is more effective if you can also keep your bunion warm with a hot water bottle. Leave the poultice on for several hours, if possible repeat once in the morning and once at night.
- A cold compress of, or soothing footbath with, five drops of German chamomile essential oil.

See the Arthritis section (p. 21) as anti-inflammatory substances that help people with arthritis may also help the inflammation of bursitis – see fish oils, GLA (in evening primrose oil and starflower oil) the herb boswellia, also the herb white willow for its anti-inflammatory and pain relieving effects, which are similar to aspirin but slower acting, longer lasting and without the side effect of gut irritation.

Note: the most helpful long-term move you can make is to ditch any bunion-inducing footwear, or only wear it for special occasions. But the toe will need looking at by a chiropodist. If the problem is really severe, daycare surgery with local anaesthetic may be needed to straighten things out.

CURRY CURE

Turmeric powder (that spice that turns Indian food yellow) and ointment containing cayenne pepper are both, despite their powerful flavours, anti-inflammatory – even though cayenne can burn a little the first couple of times. Rub some on the bunion for a while and see if it helps.

CHILDBIRTH

Childbirth is labour, the natural process by which mothers usually bring their babies into the world. On average it lasts for anything between six and twenty-four hours. First-time births are longer – an average of seven to nine hours; second and subsequent births are shorter, on average approximately four to five hours of 'true labour'. Labour has three (some would argue, four) distinct stages:

- During the first stage, the muscles of your womb are contracting with increasing strength to:
  a) shorten and 'pull up' the womb itself.
  b) open out or dilate the cervix, the lower entrance to the womb, so that your baby has a doorway to leave what has been its home for the last forty weeks.
- Next comes the transition stage (felt by many health professionals to be a brief time at the end of the first stage, although some obstetricians still refuse to admit it exists). This is when the womb's contractions change from the ones which make your womb smaller and your cervix bigger, to the strong expulsive type that actually push your baby out and down the birth canal.
- The pushing stage (some call it the 'second' stage) of labour, usually lasts between half an hour to an hour, but it can be as rapid as a few minutes or as long as two or three hours – and your baby is born at the end of it.

- Finally, the third stage is when your womb carries on contracting to gently push the placenta out through your vagina.

LABOUR – HOW WAS IT FOR YOU?

Some women find childbirth doesn't really hurt 'as such' at all, and say they were more conscious of making a huge physical effort rather than of being in pain. Others found it increasingly painful as their contractions (the clenching of the womb) became longer and closer together. Different descriptions of how it felt, taken from a survey I carried out with the help of the midwifery team, and mothers, at St George's Hospital in London, 1994 include:

- 'Familiar. It was like having sharp period pains, early on'
- 'I just thought I had bad bellyache'
- 'I really thought I had just eaten something bad – my stomach was sort of heaving and I wanted to be sick'
- 'Bad wind – I thought. Then they said I was seven centimetres dilated. I couldn't believe it'
- 'Slicing, sideswiping pains'
- 'A dull, sickening ache in my lower back'
- 'Slicing pain across my pubic area'
- 'Nothing. Had an epidural and played Scrabble for hours.'

The 'How bad did it get?' rating varied from 'not half as bad as I expected' and 'really exciting' or 'very tiring, but OK I guess' to 'excruciating' and 'no one ever told me it would be this bad'.

The pain aspect of labour tends to come from tension and from waste products building up in the womb's muscles, irritating the nerve endings there and then those muscles become short of oxygen (the squeezing keeps cutting off the blood flow). Oxygen-starved muscles hurt, as anyone who has ever had angina can tell you.

Pain signals also come from the stretching of the cervix as it

> *The pain aspect of labour tends to come from tension and from waste products building up in the womb's muscles, irritating the nerve endings there. Then those muscles become short of oxygen*

gently opens up. The other very important factor in how much pain a woman feels in labour is relaxation. Fear causes tension which causes – physiologically, never mind psychologically – more pain. If a woman is distressed or nervous during labour, the hormones this produces (like adrenaline and cortisol) affect her output of the calming and pain-soothing hormones, the endorphin group. If her endorphin output drops, she feels more pain and also begins to produce another group of hormones called catecholamines. Catecholamines do two things – affect womb contractions, and act as pain transmitters in their own right.

Yet the more relaxed you are, the more endorphins your system makes, the less you feel any pain and the more relaxed you become. This sets up a gentle circle, rather than a vicious circle. It is the tremendous power your own mind has to relax you which gives you the strongest natural weapon there is to soothe pain during childbirth.

CHILDBIRTH DOESN'T HAVE TO HURT

Most women say that they would like to try and just use natural methods of pain relief during their labours if possible. It usually is possible, as long as you have enough information beforehand about what you can do for yourself (or what your partner can do for you), the medical staff around you are supportive, and your labour is going reasonably smoothly.

Sometimes, though, things just don't go smoothly at all, despite your and everyone else's best efforts. If you find this is the case for you, you may also find that you feel it would be best to change tactics, and maybe try one or more of the medical methods of pain relief for labour every major hospital has available. These methods include powerful local painkilling drugs (epidurals work excellently for ninety-five per cent of women), the narcotic drug pethidine (about half of all women using it say it's 'good' or 'very good'), and paracervical blocks, a local anaesthetic, which may be used if you are having an assisted delivery i.e. the medical staff are using forceps or ventous suction to help your baby emerge from your birth canal. If you are exhausted by a long, too-slow labour, or if you are finding it just too painful to cope with after all, where's the shame in that? You've done the very best you possibly can. Let it go. Accepting help is a mark of strength not weakness. This isn't a bravery test or a competition, and you don't get a gold medal for going through hell without comment. So what if some other women seem to be managing OK on a bit of gas 'n' air, or by using visualisation? Or that mother of four in the next room is so relaxed and pain-free, she's fallen asleep in her birthing pool? Lucky them – but every woman handles labour differently because no two labours are ever alike. You get by the best way you can, depending on the individual circumstances.

Every single mother's labour is different, just as every woman's baby is as unique as she is herself. Labour is about mothers being treated with sensitivity and respect, having as many options as possible, choosing the best ones for themselves personally (and for their baby) under very individual circumstances. It's about what you want, and also what you find you can manage – and you cannot be certain about what you can handle and for how long, until you try.

WHAT DOES GIVING BIRTH REALLY FEEL LIKE?

- 'Massive stretching and pushing, but no pain as such.'
- 'Like a Chinese burn down there.'
- 'Like being very constipated.'
- 'As if I was trying to pass a melon out of my bowels.'
- 'A sliding feeling, like toothpaste being squeezed out of a tube.'

St George's Hospital, London 'How was it for you?' survey, 1994.

NATURAL PAIN CONTROL – DOING IT FOR YOURSELF

The following natural methods are all things you can do for yourself, or that your partner can do for you. You will not need a doctor to set them up, a nurse to inject them, or a complementary therapist such as a homeopath or acupuncturist by your side for £30 plus an hour. They are also methods you can move around with freely, and use with other methods (just don't take a TENS machine into a bath).

Many mothers have said they used certain techniques for one part of their labour, say the first few hours, then switch to heftier methods if you find you need them, for the latter half. You can team up any of the natural methods in combination with each other – reflexology and massage, breathing and acupressure. Mix and match, change over. Different methods may be suitable at different points during your labour, depending on what you feel you need and how things are going.

RELAXATION AND BREATHING

This is usually taught in ante-natal classes. But if you missed out, just try breathing in for a count of eight, holding it for eight, breathing out for eight. Try this 10-20 times. See? Your breathing has now naturally slowed and deepened. And controlling your breathing is the quickest, easiest way to reduce your heart rate, metabolic rate and to relax your muscles.

When a contraction is peaking (they start gently, build up, peak, then die away again) take a slow deep breath and 'blow' the pain away. It's simple, but it's effective – according to the National Birthday Trust (NBT) 1990 survey, eighty-nine per cent of women who used breathing control in some way said it was either a 'good', or 'very good', form of pain relief for them.

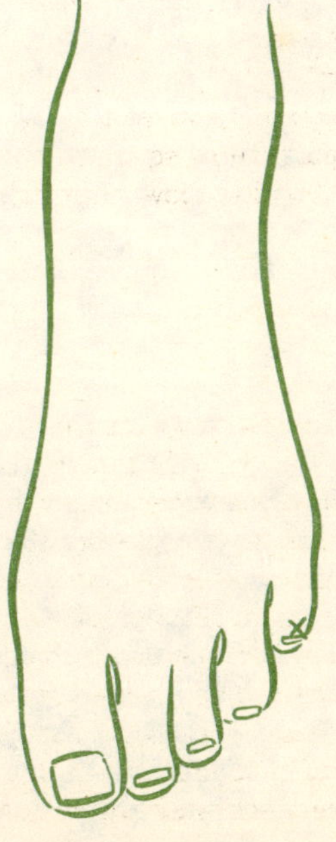

To help soothe labour pain, and encourage your womb to contract efficiently to help labour go smoothly. This is called the Zhiyan point, just outside of your little toe, by the outer corner of your toenail. Press gently but firmly using the head of a matchstick.

Note: if you're feeling very nervous or panicky, it can help greatly to take four drops of Rescue Remedy in a glass of water every fifteen to thirty minutes – or take two directly under your tongue if you're a bit beyond drinking tidily from a glass. This is the Bach Flower composite remedy for fear and panic and while not dramatic, you suddenly realise you are not feeling nearly as bad as you thought you were. Independent midwives (who are ex NHS, and now work as private practitioners) have long given Rescue Remedy to women in labour to break the vicious circle of fear/tension/pain. You can buy Rescue Remedy from most major chemist chains, and from health food shops.

WATER

A birth pool if the hospital has one or you can hire your own (see p.144). A warm bath if one is available. Even a warm shower can help at a pinch – try directing the force of hot water on your lower back if you are getting backache. There is definitely something about water that is immensely calming, and the warmth, support and light all-over pressure of it around your body are useful pain relievers.

There is no research specifically on the pain-relief power of water that I can find. However, anecdotally there are 'thousands of satisfied mothers' in the UK alone. According to leading obstetrician Dr Yheudi Gordon of the St John/St Elisabeth, and Royal Garden Hospitals in London, and active birth pioneer Janet Balaskas, both of whom are great water-birth enthusiasts: 'Being in water won't take away the pain as an epidural does – but it enhances your ability to cope by relaxing you very deeply. You are able to open up and go with your labour rather than resist it.'

THE ALTERNATIVE BIRTH BAG

Forget all those articles in glossy women's magazines which instruct you to pack designer Evian facial spray, coloured lip moisturiser ('Hospital air's so drying') stationery and stamps. New mothers say they found the following invaluable

- a vast t-shirt
- a pair of warm non-slip socks
- a Walkman and tapes
- a secret stash of chocolate/favourite biscuits/glucose tablets

- a bottle of pure water
- Rescue Remedy
- lavender essential oil
- Homeopathic Kali carb 200 for back pains and Belladonna for desperately sharp ones
- Make up a plastic bag containing equal measures of dried herbs uva ursa, comfrey and shepherds purse – put a mixed handful in your post-natal baths, and soak in it for twenty minutes for high-speed healing of sore nether regions.

For *afterwards pack*

- three pairs of baggy man's briefs
- very soft sanitary towels, such as Dr White's Maternity towels (this is no time for Always Ultra-Slims) and – forget this letter writing lark –
- a mobile phone, borrowed if necessary.

HOMEOPATHY

If you have already seen a good homeopath while you were pregnant, and explained to them that you would like to use homeopathy as a method of pain control and a way of helping your labour go smoothly, you or your partner can keep in contact with a homeopath by phone during labour, having taken a recommended birth kit of remedies in with you. Take different remedies depending on how you are feeling and how it is all progressing, or take a basic kit with you and DIY – your homeopath can advise on this, or Helios (see p. 145) supply basic kits quickly by post. This therapy is good both for helping the body to help itself in labour, and for calming you emotionally.

> Some 5 star childbirth remedies include:
> *Arnica* 30 to reduce soreness and bruising.
> *Belladonna* 30, or at a homeopath's advice, 200, to help calm very violent or painful contractions.
> *Kali carb* for painful 'back labours' where all the discomfort seems to be focused there.
> *Pulsatilla* or *Hypericum* 30 or 200 if you are upset.
> Studies such as one carried out in 1990 at the Dept. of Obstetrics and Gynaecology at Milan University found homeopathy shortened labours for first-time mums.

REFLEXOLOGY

See a good reflexologist for advice on which areas to press, then either you, or your partner can do this for you. There is a fair amount of published Russian research that suggests reflexology helped reduce pain in the first stage of labour and more studies were carried out in London's Forest Gate district with a GP and natural childbirth pioneer called Dr Gowrie Motha and the then president of the Association of Reflexologists, Mo Usher. The two women found that mothers in their study who had received ten reflexology sessions beginning mid-pregnancy, had a tenth of the number of epidurals than is usual and shorter labours by a half to one third.

MASSAGE

A quick back rub in passing does not qualify – that is more of an encouraging 'you're doing great, keep going' message from a busy passing midwife, which in today's overworked, understaffed NHS maternity wards, is usually the most you'll get. But the ten per cent of women who have 'proper' sustained lower-back massages during labour, when they wanted it (usually from their partners), said it's either a 'good' or 'very good' form of pain relief (*National Birthday Trust survey on pain relief in labour*, 1990).

For a proper lower-back massage, rub in circles on the lower back as it helps interrupt the pain signals that are shooting up your spine to be registered by the brain. Other really helpful techniques include massaging the shoulders as tension tends to collect here during labour contractions, leaving them rigid and sore; and long, firm strokes down each side of the spine with the masseur using alternate hands, extending down the thighs and hips if there is pain referred down there too. Oh – and having your buttocks kneaded firmly, as if someone was making dough, also helps.

ACUPRESSURE

Full-blown acupuncture can be so effective for childbirth that in China it is often used as a total anaesthetic block for caesarean deliveries. Doctors at the Beijing Gynaecological and Obstetric Hospital are currently performing 1000 caesareans (out of 7000 caesarean births there every year) using acupuncture.

Several studies on acupuncture for childbirth published in western medical journals suggest that from two thirds to ninety per cent of women in labour find it reduces pain. Using the right acupressure points too, such as the one shown on p. 55, you may find that it begins to help within about half an hour. Keep up the pressure treatments every hour or so throughout your labour.

Doctors at the Beijing Gynaecological and Obstetric Hospital are currently performing 1000 caesareans (out of 7000 caesarean births there every year) using acupuncture

AROMATHERAPY

More than a pretty, relaxing smell, aromatherapy has in fact been used successfully as a method of pain relief in childbirth by several maternity units, including some in Ipswich and Southampton, and at Oxford's famous John Radcliffe Hospital in 1994, where sixty-two per cent of mothers said that the oils had helped make their contractions more effective and also, to some extent, been an effective pain killer. According to Dr Vivienne Lunny, a former pathologist, and past director of Scientific Research at the Aromatherapy Organisation Council (she also trains midwives in the use of essential oils for childbirth) 'between sixty and seventy per cent of women find even some basic, sensible self-administered aromatherapy really helps. That rises to eighty-five per cent if a trained therapist or midwife who knows about essential oils is doing it.'

You can breathe the oils in having sprinkled them on to the neck of your nightgown or t-shirt, have them massaged in to your skin using a plain carrier oil (ten drops in a palmful of plain almond or even sunflower oil, massaged on and around the lower back is a very useful basic treatment), or add them to a warm bath, which will help in its own right anyway. Try ten to fifteen drops of good quality lavender (not from the Body Shop – it's not strong enough. Decent brands include Body Treats, Tisserand, Fragrant Earth, Gerrard and Neal's Yard).

Good oils for soothing labour pain are lavender (preferably the lavender angustifolia type), clary sage and chamomile. For a calming, uplifting effect try rosewood; rose, the queen of essential oils, if you can afford her; neroli; jasmine or melissa. Be guided also by whether you personally like the smell of particular oils, or not. Aromatherapy takes about thirty minutes to have an effect if it is going to.

CRAMP

Cramp occurs when certain muscles go into painful spasm. Fixed firmly in everyone's imagination is the scenario of the cramp-stricken swimmer going down for the third time – but it usually hits on dry land, and tends to be in your feet, legs and toes. It can affect your hands (as in writer's, or exam cramp) or arms. It may be extremely painful, and can last from between a few minutes to over an hour, affecting a single troublesome muscle or an entire group. Cramp is common in athletes who use these groups of muscles for long periods. Night cramps often strike elderly people, and sometimes small children (often in the calf muscles), for no apparent reason.

Cramp is the continuous clenching or contracting of a muscle/muscle group. Shortage of oxygenated blood and a build-up of muscle waste products, such as lactic acid produce the pain. Common cramp-inducers include lack of salts (perhaps after heavy sweating during exercise or fever) heavy exercise, neurological disorders, too much repetitive movement (as in RSI see p. 115) and even hardening of the arteries in the leg.

Warning: see your GP right away if you get chest cramps during or straight after exercise as it could be angina.

THE RIGHT-NOW CRAMP ACTION PLAN

Taking the 'aah' out of cramp:

- If your toes are convulsed with cramp, hold your foot in your hand and bend your toes firmly and steadily back, keeping up even pressure for a few minutes.
- If it's your calf muscles, sit down facing a wall or sofa side, jam your foot flat against it with your leg slightly bent and push, slowly and steadily. Massage the offending area with both

hands while you are doing this.

- Lay a warm hot water bottle, covered in a towel or t-shirt, against the cramping area as heat can have a very rapid soothing effect.
- Massage the Hegu 4 acupressure point – it's in the fleshy webbing between your thumb and first finger (see diagram p.23). Do this firmly but gently by rotating the ball of your thumb on the point for four or five minutes. This is a great all-round pain soother – unless the cramp is in your hands.
- Wear red. Red socks if it's cramped toes; red long johns in bed if it's your calves that spasm on cold winter nights and red fingerless leather gloves if it's typist's cramp you suffer from. Colour therapists reckon it improves the circulation.

SEXUAL CRAMP

Some women find that during sexual arousal, or immediately after orgasm, they get a 'bruising, cramp-like pain' or a 'sharp, painful spasming' in their genital area, especially their perineum, the muscular area which separates the vagina and anus. And pain every time you climax or become aroused can be enough to put even the most sensual woman off sex.

Of the women who do get sexual cramp, many say it developed after their second or third childbirth. They also report that the faster they climax, the worse the pain can be. Some gynaecologists feel that this is because the blood vessels supplying their pelvic area became dilated by the extra oestrogen your body made during pregnancy – which is normal – but never quite went back to their usual dimensions afterwards. This means you have a relatively small (i.e. usual) volume of blood flowing through permanently enlarged veins, which produces oxygen deficiency in the area and therefore pain. And oxygen shortage hurts (that's what angina is). Medical treatments include the Pill, and Provera or Danazol as they both suppress oestrogen production.

Do the scrunch

DIY treatments include warmth, relaxation exercises, visualisation – and the pelvic scrunch. Scrunching is easy, and can be pretty effective as a sexual cramp-stopper.

All you need to do is, as soon you feel the cramp beginning, clench your pelvic muscles (pretend you are stopping a bowel movement, and stopping yourself weeing, simultaneously) as hard as you can for a slow count of ten, release, then do it again. Repeat ten times. Firm self-massage around your perineal area may also help.

Scrunching can help to move any deoxygenated blood through the blood vessels a bit faster, and bring in more oxygenated blood. Also, as with pushing back cramping toes, muscular counter-pressure can also work. You can also try this preventatively immediately after making love, before it starts to hurt.

Follow this up with a warm hot water bottle on the nether regions, or a hot bath with some more self-massage (as firmly as is comfortable) around the groin and perineal area.

Note: Women who have this type of sexual cramping say that the more foreplay they have and the slower the sexual build up, the less likely it is that the cramp strikes, but that a very rapid orgasm often causes problems.

CYSTITIS

Cystitis is the inflammation of the bladder. You know you've got it if you need to pass water far more often than usual (even when the only result is a few drops) and it burns/stings when you do. You may also have some pain in your abdomen, usually a dull heavy ache, or low backache.

Cystitis is usually caused by:

- a bacterial infection
- abrasion/rubbing (hence 'bone-shaker bike' and 'sex-marathon' cystitis)
- substances which irritate the delicate tissues of your bladder and urethra eg. scented baths; drinking alcohol
- extremes of heat and cold, such as sitting on a damp, chill brick wall waiting for a bus
- other possible triggers include thrush, antibiotics, stress, and certain foods.

TAKING THE STING OUT OF CYSTITIS NOW

If you also have a low backache as a symptom, see your GP right away as this can be a sign of infection in the kidneys and this needs treating promptly with antibiotics because it can be dangerous.

- Drink as much pure, plain water as you can. Water dilutes your urine and reduces its sting, and also helps to flush out the bladder and urethral tubes leading from it.
- Lemon barley water can be soothing. The very best kind is home made: boil up 4oz barley in 600ml water with a couple of lemon slices. Strain, add honey to sweeten and keep in fridge.
- Do you like water melon? One of the traditional Chinese remedies for cystitis is sucking large slices all day.
- Keep a very clean two-pint bottle of boiled water by the loo. Pour it over your vulva, perineum and anus (front to back) as you pass water. Refill afterwards. If it hurts to do it any other way, just pee into a bidet, if you have one, with the water running; sit in enough water to cover your nether regions in the bath, or stand in the bath with the shower head spraying warm water over the area. Wash and disinfect bath/shower/bidet very well afterwards. Some women say that when out away from home they carry a bottle of water in their bag (a small plastic bottle that formerly held spring water is fine) and fill it up from the public loo basin.
- To relieve the pain try drinking a herbal tea made from one heaped teaspoon of marshmallow and one of couchgrass in a pint of water. Leave it to brew for ten minutes, then strain and drink.
- Stay off coffee, tea and alcohol until you are completely better. Anything that is a diuretic and concentrates your urine, will make peeing sting all the more.
- If the burning is really bad, sit in a warm (not hot) bath of strong chamomile tea. It's really soothing. Stay there for fifteen to twenty minutes at least – take a good magazine or book in there with you to pass the time.

GETTING RID OF IT

Note: *Any attack of cystitis lasting longer than forty-eight hours, or one associated with fever, should be brought immediately to your doctor's attention to avoid the risk of kidney infection and damage.*

- Drink cranberry juice, between one glass and two pints a day. Studies show that this helps to reduce the number of bladder bacteria by dislodging them from the organ's walls. It also contains a natural antibacterial agent (antibiotic) called hippuric acid. Most British cranberry juice has been sweetened – it is important to get an unsweetened variety. Buy cranberry concentrate and make your own, or take it in pill form without sweetener.
- Cut out alcohol and cut right back on sugary foods like biscuits, puddings and grapes. The former suppresses the immune system's ability to fight back against infection, the latter makes it harder for your white blood cells to search and destroy bacteria.
- See a clinical nutritionist (see p. 17) to check if you have any food allergies manifesting as chronic infections, such as repeated cystitis and thrush, which have been linked to allergies in many clinical studies.
- Take 1000mg of vitamin C three times daily. It's worth buying the slow-release variety if you can, so you get a constant steady supply in your system. This increases the acidity of your urine, and cystitis-inducing bugs don't like that. It also helps you fight infection generally and has an anti-inflammatory effect. Take it, if possible, with bioflavonoids, which boost vitamin C's natural effects (500–1000mg two to four times daily plus 100–500mg bioflavonoids two to four times daily).
- Proteolytic enzymes (especially bromelain) may help. One study found 'excellent' results in twenty-two per cent of cases and 'good' for seventy-eight per cent. It's usually taken on an empty stomach.
- Massage your lower back and tummy with sandalwood essential oil (ten drops in a palmful of carrier oil).
- The following homeopathic remedies may help. Homeopathic GP Dr Andrew Lockie suggests taking them every ½ hour for up to 10 hours may be helpful:

  Berberis 6c for burning pain even when not urinating
  Cantharis 30c for when you are desperate to urinate
  Staphisagria 6c for searing pain continuing after peeing.

  One medical trial reported in the British Homeopathic Journal back in 1974 stated that the remedy for what they still coyly called 'honeymoon cystitis' (can be brought on by changing sexual positions as well as a good deal of unaccustomed sex) was twice as effective as the dummy (fake) medicine they compared it against, but that even fake medication or placebo treatment seemed to sort out forty per cent of cases.

- Drink a herbal tea made from Goldenseal: place one heaped teaspoon in boiling water and steep for three minutes. Goldenseal contains an alkaloid that fights cystitis in the same way as cranberry juice.
- The herb uva ursi (bearberry), which can kill bacteria, is a treatment often used throughout Europe for this type of infection.
- Try echinacea, an anti-inflammatory which also enhances the body's own infection-fighting systems (400-1000 mg two to three times daily).

DANDELION – THE PEE-PLANT

Dandelion's always been the 'spring-clean tonic' herb, a traditional cleanser and detoxifier. It stimulates the kidneys to make more urine (the French call it *piss-en-lit* – with good reason) and cleans the liver by encouraging the gall bladder to release extra bile.

PREVENTING A RE-RUN

- Drink a couple of pints of plain, pure water daily.
- When you pee, empty your bladder completely.
- After emptying your bowels, always, always wipe from front to the back.
- Read *Cystitis* by Angela Kilmartin, (Thorsons, 1994) for the ultimate anti-cystitis regime. Try following her advice. You may never burn again.
- The herbs uva ursi (bearberry) mixed with dandelion can help prevent recurrent attacks, according to research at Sweden's Karolinska Institute in 1993. The mix is commercially available in health shops as UVA-E.
- Use small vaginal pessaries containing 500mg of the friendly bacteria lactobacillus acidophillus: use twice a week for two weeks, then once a month for two months. Research (see p.149) suggests this halves the return rate.

HOVERING AND FLEXING

Beware pee-stopping pelvic exercises ('to see how strong the love muscles are getting'). Never hover over the toilet seat when having to pass water in dubious public loos either. The former will encourage the retention of a few mls of urine in which bacteria can multiply faster than photons in a fast-breeder reactor. The latter makes your muscles tense so you don't empty your bladder properly, with the same result. Both encourage bladder re-infection. Put some loo paper over the seat instead and sit down.

EARACHE

You've got three parts to your ear: the outer, middle and inner ears. Any one of them can become infected (by a virus, fungi, or bacteria) or inflamed (piercingly cold windy winter walk – WWW – earache). The resulting earache can vary widely, from the mildly nagging to the stupendous.

Earache always needs to be checked by a GP if it's not improved substantially within twenty-four hours of self-soothing and DIY treatment for an infant or child, or forty-eight hours for an adult

Outer ears are prone to boils and abscesses. These can take the form of swimmers ear (do not clean out or scratch inside the ear with fingers after swimming off the greater proportion of British beaches, or rivers), or scratch-and-prod infections, mostly caused by the probings of sharp external objects, such as matchsticks or fingernails, which are used to remove wax balls. You've probably got an outer ear infection if it hurts to tug your ear lobe.

Middle ear infections and blockages can be caused by bacteria and viruses. The pus they produce raises the pressure inside the middle ear and this can hurt like hell. Wax blocking the ear here hurts too, but the pain usually comes on slowly. Children with glue ear may not complain that it hurts but may say, if old enough to talk, that they cannot hear you properly – it's actually like listening to someone with your fingers lightly in your ears.

Inner ear infections are usually caused by viruses and can be a legacy left over from flu, stinking colds, or diseases like mumps and measles.

Note: earache always needs to be checked by a GP if it's not improved substantially within twenty-four hours of self-soothing and DIY treatment for an infant or child, or forty-eight hours for an adult. Because there is little room for any swelling, infections can get really painful fast. And if the problem is something like an abscess, no amount of sensible at-home measures are really going to help.

SOOTHE THAT PAIN NOW

FOR ADULTS AND OLDER CHILDREN:

- Wipe a drop of German chamomile essential oil carefully around the ear to cool the area. In a palmful of carrier oil mix three drops

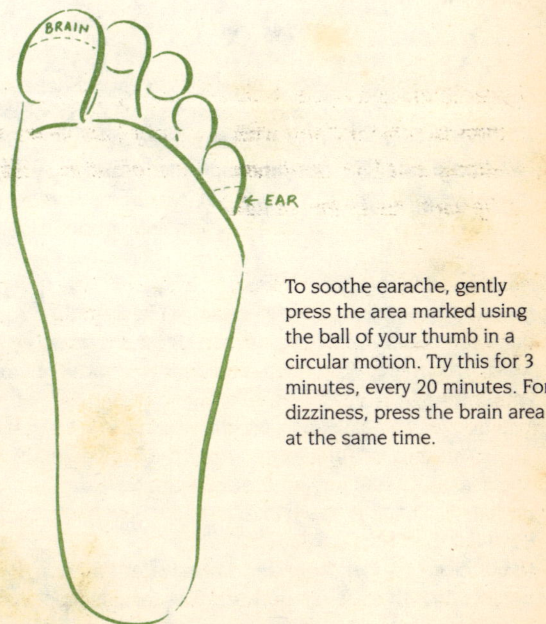

To soothe earache, gently press the area marked using the ball of your thumb in a circular motion. Try this for 3 minutes, every 20 minutes. For dizziness, press the brain area at the same time.

of lavender essential oil and two drops of tea tree, and rub around the ear area, but not in the ear, to help reduce inflammation and infection three times daily for up to three days.

- Fill a hottie, wrap in a towel or sweatshirt and place against your ear for up to 10 mins at a time (don't make the water too hot).
- Gently drip three to four drops of slightly warmed olive oil into your ear, tilting your head to one side until the oil trickles down inside. You can do the same with warmed garlic oil (pierce an ordinary garlic oil capsule) as this is also anti-infective as well as soothing and moisturising. Repeat three to four times a day, and if you wake up in pain at night. This also works well for infants and children (only use a couple of drops for them).
- Press the Hegu (Liver 4, see diagram on p. 23) acupressure point in the web of your index finger and thumb. Find the spot that's most sensitive and work it gently by rotating your thumb ball there firmly for four to five minutes at a time, with twenty minute breaks in between.

CANDLES AND COLOUR

- Colour therapists advise wrapping a green or blue scarf around your ears to soothe and cool earache inflammation. And when you lie in bed use a green or blue pillowcase too.
- Light up a candle. Hopi ear candles (approximately £4.50 a pair from selected health shops, and the homeopathic pharmacy Helios – see p. 145) are said to warm and soothe.

BABIES AND INFANTS

- Use a warm hot water bottle covered in a soft cloth. Place the child upright on your lap turned sideways against you. Slip the warm bottle between their ear and your body, holding them gently.
- Use two or three drops of warmed olive oil, or garlic oil (see above) to drip into their ears. Hold their head gently over at an angle, or lie them on their side with the ear you are treating uppermost, until it has trickled inside. Plug it gently with a soft cotton ball.
- Use a clean flannel dipped in warm water and rung out well, to hold against their ear(s). Repeat for as long as it seems to help.
- Help your child to sleep semi upright – it usually hurts worst

when they lie flat as the pressure inside the infected ear(s) builds up quickly.

- Keep the ear(s) warm by covering them with a cotton bonnet.

SUCK AWAY THE PAIN

If they are young babies, or even toddlers who still like a comfort bottle or breastfeed now and then, let them suckle. Researchers at the University of Maryland Dental School in Baltimore found in 1997 that the act of suckling can ease pain for infants because it triggers their own endorphin output. If it's a bottle, make it slightly sweet – breastmilk is – as apparently sugar boosts the pain-soothing effect.

EYESTRAIN

Computer Eye, Internet Eye, Anorak Eye, or BookWorm's Blues – they all mean eyestrain. They may not be accepted medical terms but they describe the discomfort caused by prolonged use of the eyes, and tiredness of the extra-ocular muscles which keep your eyes aligned. Symptoms include tightness around the eyes; difficulty in focusing; headaches (especially in a band across the eyes and temples) and may even translate into facial muscle pain, neck and shoulder pain especially if coupled with working at a VDU screen for long periods. Your sitting position is also a major contributing factor to muscle pain here.

Eyestrain may be provoked by watching TV for too long in the dark; working in very bright or very dim light; long periods of reading or close work and wearing the wrong prescription glasses; and fluorescent lights because of the frequency at which they flicker.

THE FIVE-MINUTE ANTI-EYESTRAIN WORKOUT

This workout is easy, very relaxing, and based on acupressure.

1. Shut your eyes and block out the computer screen if you are working on one.
2. Using your index finger and thumb, massage the top of the nose bridge in an up and down movement for one to two minutes.
3. Place your index fingers on the inner corner of your eyebrows, so that you can feel the ridge of bone below. Push down and slide fingers outwards in opposite directions to the end of the eyebrows, then continue the finger-pressure stroke round the eye socket's bony rim, along the temples and curling around the ears. Repeat three to five times.
4. Using your knuckle to press against your forehead between the eyebrows, around where yoga pictures of the third eye are (and a centimetre or so upwards for some people – feel around till you find the sensitive area – bingo, that's the spot you press). Lean the weight of your head gently against the knuckle, bone on bone, for a minute or so. This stimulates the acupressure spot called Yintang, and it also helps soothe headaches caused by tight neck and shoulder muscles, and is very calming and centring generally.
5. Keep your eyes closed for at least a minute. Open them slowly focusing first on something distant for ten seconds, then on a close object, before resuming work/reading/TV watching.

FINGERNAIL POWER

Hold up your fourth finger (doesn't matter which hand) and mentally draw a square grid to enclose the nailbed and nail (see diagram p. 95). See the points in each of the lower corners of the box you have sketched? These are the finger medial and lateral nail points of acupressure. Stimulate them gently for a minute or two at a time with the nail edge of one of the fingers of your other hand to produce a painkilling effect for aching eyes.

COLOUR THERAPY CURE

Lie with your eyes shut. Place light blue eyepads that have been soaked in cool water on your eyes for ten minutes. Or, look towards, without particularly focusing on, anything cool green (trees, grass) for a few minutes.

REJUVENATING TIRED, STRAINED EYES

- Place thin slices of cucumber from the fridge on your eyes.
- Make a herbal decoction of euphrasia (country people call it eyebright), chickweed or marigold. Cool the mixture, soak eyepads made from cotton wool in it, wring out and place over your eyes. To make a decoction: use one ounce of the dried herb to 1.1 pints of water, bring to the boil in a saucepan (not an aluminium one), cover and simmer for fifteen minutes. Strain, cool rapidly in a fridge/freezer, then use.
- Mother tincture of euphrasia (from a homeopathic pharmacy – a lot less trouble than boiling up your own herbal brew). Put four drops in a quarter of a pint of warm water and bathe your eyes. Some clued-up national journalists and bond traders even keep a bottle of this euphrasia tincture in their desk at work they need it so often – next to the bumper bottle of Bach Flower Rescue Remedy.

Do you have eyeache as a result of too much sex? Homeopaths say this can happen – and even recommend a special remedy for it – Phosphorous 6c

- Be your own homeopath.
  Homeopathic GP Dr Andrew Lockie suggests the following may be helpful:
  Arnica 6c if your eyes are strained from looking into the distance for long periods. Take 4 times daily for up to 7 days.
  Ruta 6c if they are strained from reading for long periods or close work. Take 4 times daily for up to 7 days.

SEXY EYES

Do you have eyeache as a result of too much sex? Homeopaths say this can happen – and even recommend a special remedy for it – Phosphorous 6c.

FIRST AID: CUTS, GRAZES, BITES, BRUISES, SPRAINS, BURNS, SCALDS AND SUNBURN

BITES AND STINGS FROM INSECTS

Insect bites and stings pierce the protective outer layers of your skin and can cause swelling, redness or infection. Some simply itch a bit – others can throb, burn and sear for days, depending on what bit you and how your system reacts to its particular venom. Of all the local winged biters, horseflies are probably the most painful.

Bees leave their sting and its attached venom sac behind, and often you can see it clearly protruding from the skin. Scrape it away with a sharp knife (if you've got one handy) or the edge of a credit card, then tweezer out the sting itself, which looks like a hair-fine splinter. Don't try to squeeze the sac out as this may burst it, forcing the bee's venom into the surrounding skin. Wasp stings don't leave venom sacs behind, so just tweeze out the sting.

Mosquitoes leave no calling card either apart from a reddening lump. Britain's hot summer of 1997 offered bumper mozzie conditions, which produced a lot more of the insects than usual. Some of them appeared to be a particularly vicious type which left bites that spread in many cases until they were inches across and weeping clear fluid from the bite site itself. These may remain miserably itchy and painful for two or three days. Rubbing on a few drops of essential oil of lavender (especially wrists, ankles, tips of ears, collarbone and a dab down the cleavage, and elbow/knee creases) may help act as a mosquito repellent.

STINGER ALERT

There is a very rare, but potentially life-threatening, reaction to being bitten/stung called anaphylactic shock. Symptoms can include nausea, feeling dizzy and faint, troubled breathing and a fast, weak pulse. Dial 999, and stay with the person, being as reassuring as you can but not moving them or giving them anything to eat or drink, until the ambulance arrives.

TAKING THE STING OUT OF AN INSECT BITE

Soothing things to dab on to the bite:

- Ice cubes: rub gently
- Bach Flowers Rescue Remedy: put four drops in half a cup of water
- Iced water with baking soda (strong enough to taste it)
- Marigold (calendula) ointment
- Lavender essential oil
- Undiluted homeopathic mother tinctures – *Pyrethrum* is a good general one, but specifics include:
  Ledum for bee stings
  Arnica or *ledum* for hornets and wasps
  Hypericum and *calendula* mixed together if you've been set upon by a cloud of midges on a hot, sultry summer evening
- Plain pure aloe vera gel may be soothing if rubbed on gently

Rubbing on a few drops of essential oil of lavender may help act as a mosquito repellent

HOMEOPATHIC HELP

Apis 30 if it swells rapidly, is red and really itchy
Cantharis 30c if it's red and burning
Tarentula (*sic*) 6c if its bluish and burning.

There is also a German homeopathic after-bite gel called *Prrikweg* (and yes it is spelt that way) with which the London School of Hygiene and Tropical Medicine has carried out successful trials.

BRUISES

Bruises can be tender to the touch or they may cause a deep aching, throbbing pain at the site of the injury. A good bruise will bloom characteristically black and purple whenever the body

To soothe a bad bruise and help it to heal faster, take vitamin C (1000-2000*mg three times a day*)

receives an impact blow hard enough (whether it's catching your thigh on the corner of a table or falling off a motorbike) to break open some of the blood capillaries which weave and thread through the body's soft tissues.

Bruising happens especially easily if a component of the blood clotting process is missing, as with haemophilia. Deep bruising can take three or four days to appear on the surface of the skin and can be particularly painful until it 'comes out'. When you are short of vitamin C, you tend to bruise more easily as it is thought to be vital for the formation of collagen, the elastic substance that keeps blood vessel walls flexible and strong.

Note: if bruising has not cleared up within two weeks or appears for no apparent reason, go to your GP and have it checked out.

SOFTENING THE BLOW OF BRUISING

If you have badly bruised an arm or leg, you do need to rest it for twenty-four to forty-eight hours, preferably raised up on supportive soft pillows, to lessen blood flow to the area while the capillaries are knitting themselves back together.

To soothe the pain and encourage rapid healing:

- Take vitamin C, up to 1000mg three times a day if you are smaller with a light frame or up to 2000mg three times a day if you are heavier with a tall frame.
- Use a herbal rosemary compress, warm or cool on the area, whichever is the most soothing. Pour half a pint of boiling water onto 1-2 tbsp of dried rosemary, or 3 tbsp of fresh rosemary. Leave to stew for 20 minutes. Soak a flannel in the brew, wring out and wrap gently around the affected area while still hot. Leave for 10 minutes.
- Add in some drops of lavender essential oil as this discourages inflammation in the area, too, so it will hurt less.
- Use *arnica*, as an ointment or add tincture of *arnica* to half a glass of cool water and dip a clean flannel into this, using it as a cool, healing compress; or take it by mouth as homeopathic *arnica* 30*c* pills or powders. Take four daily for up to three days.

BE YOUR OWN HOMEOPATH

Work carried out at the University of Nantes in France in 1981 found a mix of *apis* and *arnica* was useful for bringing down the sometimes impressive swelling and bruising patients develop when they have had jaw or facial surgery. Alternatively, try:

Hypericum 30*c* if it's your fingers or toes you've bruised (perhaps stubbed your toe badly or slammed your fingers in a door)

Ruta 6*c* if it's really deep bruising that feels like it's on a bone

Bellis 6*c* if you have had a blow on the breast.

Take these remedies four times daily for up to three days. If no improvement, see your GP, as your bruising might need further investigation.

SPRAINS AND STRAINS

Sprains are ligament injuries. Ligaments are the strong, fibrous strings which help to hold a joint together. They can tear when twisted or wrenched, causing pain which can vary from uncomfortable to excruciating, when you abruptly stretch or turn beyond your usual range of movement. Signs of a sprain include swelling, stiffness, bruising and pain and it can be quite difficult in some cases to tell what's a sprain and what's a fracture, especially with a small child who has broken one of the many small bones making up their hand or foot. The general rule is 'if you can use the joint – just – it's unlikely to be broken' but if in any doubt at all, go to casualty and ask for an x-ray as there may be a small crack in the bone instead, and so the area may still need to be put in protective plaster so it can heal. If after using self help methods for three days it's no better, go and see your GP.

Ordinary self help for a sprain is the RICE (rest, ice compresses, compression binding and elevation) system, much used in sports injury but a good, practical DIY recipe for soothing a sprain from any source. The *Rest* bit is usually for twenty-four to forty-eight hours; *Ice* means put on a pack of crushed ice or frozen peas/sweetcorn wrapped in a soft cloth immediately before the area starts to swell; *Compression* means supporting the injury comfortably in a Tubigrip style bandage; *Elevation* means putting the injured area up, and if it's an arm or shoulder, using a sling support.

INSTANT HOMEOPATHIC FIRST AID

Take *Arnica* 30*c* tablets, four times daily for three days to reduce bruising and swelling – Guys and St Thomas Trust in London often suggest *arnica* for plastic surgery patients to reduce swelling after their operations.

TO RUB ON

- *Bach Flowers Rescue Remedy cream*
- *Arnica or calendula cream*, better still a mix of both (you can get these in any health shop and many independent chemists). One of the new Continental sports-injury rubs, made in Germany – Traumeel S – contains arnica, calendula, hamamelis, millefolium and minute amounts of mercury and sulphur. It is widely used in specialist sports injury clinics there, and in one huge trial of 3,422 patients suffering from tenosynovitis (RSI) haematomas, sprains and strains, ninety-eight per cent found the results very good/good/satisfactory.
- *Lavender essential oil* (can help reduce inflammation and may also have an analgesic (pain killing) effect.
- A *homeopathic compress*: if you are putting on a cooling compress, add some drops of homeopathic *arnica* tincture to the water for extra effect.

SPORTS TIP – STOP ACHING MUSCLES

If you are about to make a major physical effort – whether its childbirth, a racquet game you're dreading against someone a lot better than you, or even running a half marathon – and expect to be really sore and aching afterwards, take vitamin C preventatively and your muscles will hurt far less. Dosage: approx 3,000 mgs (taken in three 1,000mg doses morning, afternoon and evening) for ten days before a major sporting event.

CUTS AND GRAZES

Cuts and grazes are usually minor and it's generally just the capillaries which are damaged, causing small amounts of blood to be released in the surrounding tissues, or to bleed from the wound itself. The wound clots rapidly and does not require much treatment. However, even small cuts can be painful especially if they are relatively deep (like paper cuts). Grazes tend to be disproportionately sore to the amount of actual damage that has been done, as any parent of small children could confirm.

Calendula is homeopathy's top remedy for healing cuts and wounds

Grazes need to be cleaned with cool clean water, and if necessary a loose lint dressing can be put on to protect them for a day or so. Clean cuts the same way then press gently but very firmly on them to stop the blood flowing. A severe cut may need stitches or some medical 'skin glue' to help it heal well.

If a small child has even a relatively minor cut that is still bleeding and really sore, put a drop of neat lavender oil on a plaster and cover it up. After it's clotted, take off the plaster and expose the area to fresh air (if the child won't let you near it, do this gently at night when they are asleep). Try homeopathic *Hypericum* ointment if the cut is causing a lot of pain. Calendula is homeopathy's top remedy for healing cuts and wounds: bathe the area in a warm solution of one cup (240ml) of pre-boiled, cooled water and one teaspoon of calendula tincture.

Note: wounds and cuts with a good deal of dirt in them, or which you cannot completely clean yourself at home, need to be cleaned by a nurse. If soil has got into or around the cut/graze, check that you or your child are up to date with tetanus jabs. All children should be vaccinated against tetanus.

BURNS AND SCALDS

Burns are caused by dry heat (such as electricity, strong sunlight, fire or chemicals). *Scalds* are produced by damp heat, such as boiling water from a kettle, or steam. The effect both have on your skin is the same – painful tissue damage. Even a small burn/scald can really hurt. With mild or first-degree burns the damage is limited to the top layers of skin. The area will redden up, feel hot, very sore and possibly blister as well. These can hurt like hell but are seldom serious unless they cover a large area of your skin. Second-degree burns are more serious because the heat damage has gone deeper, damaging the lower layers of your skin and blistering. Third-degree burns are very serious because they reach the living flesh under the skin. If you have either a second- or a third-degree burn you will probably also go into shock.

First-degree burns (such as sunburn, or when you've caught your arm on a hot saucepan) you can usually treat yourself at home, as long as they are not too big, but if they do not feel more comfortable within twenty-four to forty-eight hours, see your doctor. Anything more serious means going to casualty right away.

IMMEDIATE ACTION TIPS

- If it's a burn rather than a scald, bathe it in cold water for ten to fifteen minutes, or hold it under a gently running cold tap for the same amount of time. Then cover lightly with a clean, non-fluffy bandage or cloth.
- A minor burn or scald? Drip a few drops of undiluted essential oil of lavender over the area.
- Upset, shocked? Take four drops of Rescue Remedy in a half glass of water. Sip slowly.
- For minor burns, put aloe vera gel on them as long as the skin's not broken; if it is, use calendula cream instead.
- If your burn scars are painful, take homeopathic *Causticum* 6 four times daily for seven days.

DAMAGE-LIMITATION

- Burns/scalds: every fifteen minutes take up to three doses of Homeopathic *Arnica* 30, followed by up to six doses of *Cantharis* 30. You can do this in conjunction with orthodox medical treatment if the burns are second- or third-degree too, but it is safest to wait until after the burn has been cooled and you have called a doctor or ambulance.
- Take 1g of vitamin C three–four times a day to help rapid healing, for up to two days. Try to get the slow-release type (ask at the healthfood shop or at a major chemist for the available types) so your body maintains a good level of it in the system all the time.
- If the burn/scald carries on stinging, try *Urtica* 6, for up to six doses.

SUNBURN

Painful in the short term, sunburn can do lasting damage long term, as the link between sunburn, rapidly ageing skin and skin cancer, is now inescapable. If you want a bit of a tan, get a very slight skin-warmer rather than a mahogany makeover. Take it very slowly over several weeks and top up with fake tan mixed equally with moisturiser so it doesn't streak and give you stripey legs.

PULL AWAY THE PAIN

A good DIY acupressure first-aid trick for soothing sunburn is to massage both ear lobes, pulling them down slightly as you do so; and massage the bridge of your nose (as long as it's not too sore to touch).

The Australian sunwatch publicity campaign basically says it all, for both children and adults 'Slip, Slop, Slap' – slip on a baggy covering t-shirt, slop on a high factor sun protection cream or total sunblock and slap on a shady hat. This goes double for children and babies. Their delicate skin is easily burnt by sun so their slop component needs to be a total sunblock, preferably water resistant and their t-shirts long sleeved if possible, or at least with sleeves covering the top of their shoulders – vest-style t-shirts are not much use.

Again (and you'll have heard this often before but it doesn't make it any less true) for everyone who wants to save their skin, stay out of the 11am to 3pm sun. On holiday, take a siesta for languid sex and sleep, go to the bar, have a really long holiday lunch, let the children play on covered verandahs or inside (a good reason to take kids' videos on holiday and ask for a video machine in villas or to go to a child-friendly holiday centre with an indoor children's club or big covered play area). If you do hit the pool, wear a sunhat and t-shirt – UV light goes through water. It also goes through cloud, so a grey day means you can still get badly burnt.

HOW TO TAKE THE STING OUT OF SUNBURN

Emergency measures;

- Used, cold tea bags, or better still really stewed tea from the morning's breakfast if it's still in the teapot, to wipe over burnt areas. Put in the freezer for a few minutes first if possible. Tea contains tannic acid, which is anti-inflammatory.
- Cut a cucumber into thin slices and lay over the sunburn. Very cooling. Again, put the cucumber in the freezer for five to ten

minutes first.

- Bathe in a bath of just-warm water. You can also add up to ten drops of essential oil of lavender, or bicarbonate of soda so you can just taste it in the water.
- If it's a small area, such as a forearm that got 'left' in the sun (often happens when driving on holiday) immerse it in really cool water for two to three minutes at intervals. Add enough vinegar so you can just taste it.

Vinegar is a traditional anti-sting remedy for sun overdosers

- Other good small-area soothers: calendula (marigold) ointment; hypericum (St Johns Wort) oil or ointment; Rescue Remedy cream or vitamin E cream. Keep the tubes/pots in the fridge so they are very cool when needed.
- Apply cold yoghurt straight out of the fridge. Leave it on for as long as is comforting before rinsing it away with lukewarm water from the shower head, and wiping clean gently.
- Make an infusion of chamomile flowers by steeping two teaspoons in a cup of boiling water for ten minutes. Chamomile tea bags steeped in boiling water for 10-15 minutes will do at a pinch. Dip a pad of cotton wool into the *cooled* tea, soak it and use this to gently wipe the sunburned area, re-wetting the cotton wool in the chamomile solution as often as you need to.

Note: If the person also has a fever, if the sunburn is also blistered, or is not calming down within twenty-four hours for a child or forty-eight hours for an adult – seek prompt medical advice.

FLU AND FEVER

Technically you have a fever if your body temperature goes above normal (i.e. 96.8-98.6 F or 36-7C). In reality, a degree or two F won't make you feel much worse, but higher fevers can really make you ache from head to foot. Fevers are usually caused by bacterial or viral infections such as colds, chickenpox, flu, measles, cystitis, pelvic infections, tonsillitis and gastroenteritis.

Temperatures, though most people tend to swat them pretty sharpish with aspirin (Calpol if the fever's broken out in an infant) are actually goods news, because they are a sign that your body is fighting an invading infection. They are also actually useful – and necessary – because they are the body's natural way of killing off the offending germs. Flatten a fever too soon or too much and you may be ill for longer, as the germs and the toxins they are producing, stay in your system for longer. A good time to bring a temperature down a little is at night, so you can get some decent, comfortable sleep, but you may get better faster if you do not take too much fever-reducing medication during the day.

However, a fever can also make you feel as if you have been beaten up, so badly do you ache. A decent compromise between lying in bed stoically aching and sweating, and taking fever-suppressing medication in handfuls at the first drop of perspiration, is to:

1. Boost your immune system immediately.
2. Drink (plain water) like a fish to encourage the elimination of toxins which the bug you have caught is producing.
3. Bring the fever down a little, rather than eliminating it altogether. It can still do its work but you don't feel quite so dreadful.

Note: if your fever stays high for more than twenty-four hours (for a child) to forty-eight hours (for an adult) no matter what you do, or if you have other symptoms, e.g. those of cystitis or gastroenteritis, call your GP right away for advice.

DRINK AWAY FEVER

- The best fever-soothing herbal teas are limeflower, chamomile, elderflower, marigold, borage and yarrow. You can use them singly, or in combination. If you find they taste boring or too sharp, add a teaspoon of honey. All the teas are made with one pint of boiling water to 1oz of the dried herb. Sadly, herbal tea bags may be convenient but they are not much good for medicinal purposes. Let the brew you have made stand for ten minutes, then strain. Drink it as often as you can. This is especially helpful if you have a raging sore throat as well.
- Make drinks of lemon and honey, or blackcurrant cordial with

boiling water. Sip on and off all day.

- Treat fever aches and pains with willow extract, which has a similar effect to aspirin but without the side effects of gut irritation.
- Drink as much pure plain water as you can in between the medicinal teas.

SELF-HELP: COLOUR ME COOLER

Greens and blues are cooling, healing colours. Try and make up your bed with sheets/pillowcases and duvet covers in these shades – colour therapists claim this can help bring down temperatures. Avoid red bed covers and pillows if you have a fever.

Be your own homeopath. These remedies and dosages are also safe for children. Take every hour for up to 10 hours, some suggestions from homeopathic GP Dr Andrew Lockie include:

Gelsenium 6c if you're feeling fluey, shivery with aching muscles and heavy eyelids, got a headache which feels worse when you move and just not thirsty despite your temperature.

Aconite 30c if your fever came on suddenly, is worse around midnight, you are thirsty, feeling restless but you are pale in the face.

Belladonna 30c if the fever came on suddenly, your skin's hot and flushed and you are a bit delirious.

TURBO CHARGE YOUR IMMUNE SYSTEM

As soon as you begin to ache from an impending fever, flu or cold, take:

Vitamin C

You've heard it before, but twenty-one placebo-controlled clinical studies can't all be wrong (see pp. 150-51) and researchers have found vitamin C cuts back the length of a cold and the nastiness of its symptoms (including a temperature and aching) by an average of twenty-three per cent. Take 1000mg three times daily until you are feeling better.

Echinacea

Available in ranges like FSC's Herbcraft in a tincture form you can just add to water and gulp down, and it's been heavily researched in Germany since the 1930s. Echinacea backs up the immune system in general by upping the activity and production rate of infection-fighting white blood cells, and it also increases your production of interferon, a vital part of the body's response to colds and flu. Dosage varies depending on how concentrated the product is, but fifteen to twenty drops of its liquid form four times daily is about average.

Greens and blues are cooling, healing colours. Try and make up your bed with sheets/pillowcases and duvet covers in these shades. Avoid red ones

Garlic

Garlic is a general broad-spectrum anti-infective agent (i.e. it kills bacteria, viruses and fungal infections with equal enthusiasm). Take 900mg per day if it's just garlic (5000mcg of its active ingredient allicin). If you don't fancy chewing fresh garlic cloves, take the specially coated 'odour-controlled' tablets available in all health food shops.

CHILDREN'S FEVER ALERT

Any temperature over 102F or 39C can be dangerous for an infant or child, so always telephone your GP for advice. If their temperature remains at 102F for six hours or more, call immediately for emergency treatment. Cool your child down by covering them in just a cotton sheet, and, exposing one limb at a time only, sponge them down with warm (not cold) water. If you have any essential oil of lavender, Roman chamomile or pettigran use three drops per basinful of water.

Never, ever, put a feverish child in a cold bath as it could send them into shock. If the sponging alone isn't enough, use infant paracetamol (like Calpol) in the relevant dose. If you see signs of an impending fit (febrile convulsions) brought on by the sudden increase in their temperature,

Never, ever, put a feverish child in a cold bath as it could send them into shock

sponge them down to cool them if there is time. If there clearly isn't, get under a lukewarm shower with them right away, fully clothed if necessary. This produces rapid cooling which should head off the convulsions.

HEADACHES AND MIGRAINES

MIGRAINES (VASCULAR HEADACHES)

Migraines are very powerful and painful headaches, involving a severe throbbing pain which always begins (and often stays) on one side of the head. Conservative estimates suggest one in ten of us have migraines, but the British Migraine Association reckons it's nearer one in five for men, up to one in every three women, and in half of all cases the problem runs in the family. Ten per cent of children may also be migraineurs, which will often show up as 'sick headaches', but they often go unrecognised. The word migraine comes from the Latin words hemi (half) and crania (head).

This is no ordinary, vicious one-sided headache. People experiencing a Classic Migraine will often feel sick, may even be sick, find it hurts just to look at ordinarily bright light or to move about, and about half will have visual disturbance warning symptoms, known as 'auras' just before the pain hits. These auras can include blurring, vision loss, seeing objects as either bigger or smaller than they really are, sparkling lights or dramatic zig zag lines like a TV screen picture sliced up by weather interference. These symptoms generally last a few minutes, and a migraineur may also find their thinking is disturbed or confused, that they are panicky, tired and dizzy.

There is also the Common Migraine, where severe or warning symptoms are rare, and the severe throbbing may be on one/both sides of the head and last for anything between one and three days; or the Cluster Headache. This is the least common type of all and involves severe pain usually just around one eye. It has no warning symptoms, may be linked to sensitivity to light, crying tears, even a stuffed up nose and tends to happen in clusters of between one and three headaches a day, continuing the pattern for several days. Once classed as a type of migraine (and often still mentioned in the same breath) specialist doctors have reclassified cluster headaches separately and now call them histaminic cephalgia, Horton's headache, or atypical facial neuralgia.

Migraine pain is caused by the shrinking and swelling of the blood vessels in the head, which cause a restricted bloodflow to the brain

Migraine pain is caused by the shrinking and swelling of the blood vessels in the head, which cause a restricted bloodflow to the brain. According to consultant neurologist Dr Shreyas Patel, medical director of The Marino Center's Pain and Stress Reduction Program in Boston USA, nerve inflammation is another very important factor. The constriction/dilation of these blood vessels is partly related to a neurotransmitter (a chemical which helps transmit electrical nerve signals) called serotonin which occurs naturally within the body. Too much or too little of this may trigger migraines.

Apart from powerful painkillers during an attack, the approaches which seem to help migraine most are:

1. Preventing another attack – there are many sensible, practical DIY measures, such as finding your own personal migraine triggers – and complementary medicine treatments that you can carry out for yourself, under the prevention umbrella.
2. Long-term maintenance treatments, such as the herb feverfew, or nutritional supplements such as magnesium.

WOMEN, HORMONES AND MIGRAINE

Pregnancy often makes migraines (temporarily) better – about seventy per cent of expectant mothers find their migraines are milder or even that they disappear altogether after the first three months. However, pregnancy seems a drastic solution and the benefit is temporary – it can make migraines worse. Migraines are often worse in the last few days before women's periods begin. Strict research trials suggest magnesium may help here.

HELPING YOURSELF

It's now well accepted that intolerances or allergies to certain foods are major migraine-triggers. The link is that allergic reactions to food cause serotonin and histamine to be released in your body, and this affects the blood flow to your brain. Some research studies say there is a food connection for as many as nine out of ten migraineurs, others say it's three out of ten. Whichever is right, what you eat is usually within your control, so it's worth a try.

THE MIGRAINE-MAKERS TOP TWENTY – AND WHAT TO EAT INSTEAD

There are various ways that the food you eat can trigger a migraine – two of the most common are allergic reaction and oversensitivity. One seminal study in the Lancet in 1983 states that the top four most common foods to have allergies to are cow's milk and anything made from it (i.e. dairy products), eggs, chocolate, and wheat products (bread, pasta). Food allergy can start a migraine because it causes the chemicals like histamine and serotonin to be released into the body.

Oversensitivity is not the same as an allergy. It means that you react more powerfully to substances than most. An oversensitivity to a group of chemicals called vaso-active amines, which are also found in food can be a trigger. Vaso-active means that they affect the diameter of your blood vessels, and therefore the amount of blood flowing through them, which can trigger off migraine attacks. The group of chemicals includes serotonin (again), tryptamine, tyramine and dopamine.

Pregnancy often makes migraines (temporarily) better – about seventy per cent of expectant mothers find their migraines are milder or even that they disappear altogether after the first three months. However pregnancy seems a drastic solution and the benefit is transitory

The suggestions below are based on a successful anti-migraine eating plan, devised by the American Council for Headache Education, called, optimistically, ' The Headache Free Diet' (1990).

AVOID:

- fresh home made yeast breads, pizza, doughnuts
- eat little citrus fruit, especially bananas, strawberries, mangoes and kiwi fruit
- avoid most cheese (see p. 89)
- tartrazine
- rye
- rice
- soy sauce
- pork
- alcohol (especially red wine so go for white and spritzers)
- monosodium glutamate (watch out for Chinese takeaway)
- Nutrasweet
- chocolate
- mincemeat
- all caffeine – that's coffee, colas and tea
- certain nuts
- oats
- cane sugar
- yeast (bad news for those who like yeast extract spreads such as Marmite on their toast – try sesame spread or Bovril)
- bacon and ham, salamis and sausages
- beans – broad, baked (fava) beans, soy beans, lentils, aubergine, spinach, tomatoes.

TRY INSTEAD:

- milk
- rice cakes
- instead of wheat-based bread or commercial breads (i.e. anything wrapped in a cheery plastic wrapper), try English muffins, pasta and rice (American experts reckon they are OK), bagels
- white wine instead of red
- an Indian, rather than Chinese, take away

- chicory coffee rather than real coffee
- carob chocolate or Caramac rather than plain chocolate (milk chocolate is reportedly less of a trigger than plain, if you hate both alternatives)
- soft drinks such as 7-Up, Sprite and ginger ale
- fruit juice (not citrus – go for apple juice, mango, guava, blackcurrant, cranberry, etc)

Some studies suggest that low-protein diets can help to cut back migraine attacks

- yeast-free biscuits and cakes; available at most decent health food shops
- sesame spread or even Bovril if you want something savoury on your toast rather than Marmite
- Quorn (fungi-protein. Use in pies or stir fry. It tastes remarkably like chicken; can be a bit dry and tastes nicest if marinated in milk for a few minutes before cooking with it.)
- sugar that's come from sugar beet rather than cane sugar, or use honey as a sweetener (not aspartame – that's also implicated in some migraines)
- use herbs, black pepper and lemon juice as flavouring rather than salting food
- some studies also suggest that sometimes low-protein diets can really help to cut back migraine attacks. To find one that you would actually enjoy living off, it's well worth going to see a nutritionist if this idea appeals because they can work out something especially for you. (For how to find a good, professional nutritionist, see the entry for the British Dietetic Assoc., in Helplines p. 143)

Note: the American Headache Free Diet is used by many headache specialists, including Dr Shreyas Patel, and it has been put together on the basis that the foods are low in tyramine (the vaso-active amino acid which can trigger migraine). However, it does differ from the British Migraine Association's dietary suggestions, which suggest no milk, no ordinary wheat-based bread either (rye bread or alternative), and no rice and potatoes. So you may need to experiment by leaving out for a week, then including back in, these major food groups and see how your system personally responds to see what works best for you on an individual basis.

Ideally it should be possible to be clinically tested accurately for food allergy – but generally speaking the tests are both expensive and often inaccurate as well. A.K. or Applied Kinesiology muscle testing may be helpful here – contact the Institute of Complementary Medicine.

WHICH CHEESE?

If cheese is something that sets you off (probably because of its tyramine content – tyramine is an amino acid which is converted to serotonin) try cottage cheese instead, because it comes bottom of the migraine-potential league, followed by medium-fat cheese and quark – feta, Brie, Camembert, Edam and Gouda are in the middle. English 'country' cheeses like Double Gloucester or Wensleydale are near the top, with the biggest culprits being Cheddar and Parmesan.

WHAT ELSE TO TAKE:

- Fish oils, possibly because the EPA and DHA (types of essential fatty acids) it contains affect the hormone-like substances called prostaglandins – however, beware the 'fishy burps' syndrome with this. There is also a possibility of tummy upsets/nosebleeds.
- Lactase supplements before you eat any dairy products like ice cream, milk shakes, milk puddings or cheeses.
- Magnesium supplements, which may be especially helpful for younger women who have not yet had their menopause.
- Hefty doses of calcium and vitamin D (800mg calcium and 400iu vit D daily).
- Ginger for migraines with sickness – ginger is a very old anti-nausea remedy and even helps up to eighty per cent of women with pregnancy morning sickness.
- Ginko Biloba extract.
- Feverfew. This herb has been used to relieve migraine for centuries but scientists have only recently found out how it works. Apparently it contains a natural chemical called parthenolide which inhibits serotonin release,

In 1988 trials at Nottingham University found that migraineurs who take feverfew had twenty-five per cent fewer attacks and suffered less nausea

and therefore encourages a more even blood flow. Clinical trials at the City of London Migraine Clinic found that seventy per cent of patients said the herb helped, and in 1988 trials at Nottingham University found that migraineurs who take feverfew had twenty-five per cent fewer attacks and suffered less nausea or vomiting during the ones they still experienced.

- Homeopathic remedies. One double-blind controlled study in Verona, Italy (1991) showed remedies such as belladonna, ignatia, silicia, gelsenium and sulphur reduced both the number and severity of attacks. Speak to a qualified homeopath about the right remedy for you personally because if you do take the wrong one it will be of no use at all.

Herb and sugar sandwiches

The British Migraine Association (BMA) recommends eating whole leaves of the feverfew plant, either fresh (many sufferers grow it in the garden – but if you do too, make sure it's the Tanacetum Parthenium or wild feverfew variety) or dried, in a sandwich sprinkled with sugar to mask the bitter taste. According to the Association, if you take it in tea format it's difficult to assess the strength of the dose. A preventative dose is two to three small leaves (measuring four centimetres by three centimetres). You can also get feverfew in tablet form which tastes far better. According to the Canadian Health Authorities, the effective daily dose is 0.2 per cent Parthenolide for each 125mg feverfew leaf powder – check any brand you buy offers this.

Note: possible side effects include mouth ulcers and skin itchiness; if you get these it may mean that feverfew isn't for you.

Which helps the most?

According to a recent survey by the British Migraine Association, migraine sufferers who opted for complementary therapies found that the herb feverfew was the most use, closely followed by acupuncture (try the DIY acupressure point shown on p. 94) and then homeopathy.

Do:

- Eat regularly, at least every four hours. Research suggests that migraines can attack when your blood sugar is low because you're hungry. Try carrying a stash of glucose tablets in your bag or

When a migraine strikes try resting your head on a frozen hot water bottle kept in readiness in the freezer

pocket if you know you've got a food gap (a long meeting or journey) coming up, or keep them there all the time for emergencies.

- Wear sunglasses that react to light. Dark lenses may be better than medium-shade ones – try ski and watersports specialist shops or store departments for some very dark ones which have an impressive record at screening out UVA, UVB and glare and have especially cool designs. Or try the wraparound variety which lets no light in around the sides – Solarshield UK make them (from Station Road Industrial Estate, Hemyock, EX15 3SE, Devon for about £18.50, including p and p).
- Try to reduce your stress levels with regular relaxation methods such as breathing/visualisation, yoga classes or home practice, meditation and/or swimming.

Note: always see your GP in the first instance if you suffer from migraine headaches, especially if they begin suddenly and out of the blue.

WHEN A MIGRAINE HEADACHE STRIKES TRY:

- A frozen hot water bottle. Many people find something cold on their head helps during an attack. Half fill an ordinary rubber hottie and keep it in the freezer, slip it under your pillow case and rest your head on it as needed. When it thaws a bit it is soft enough to go to sleep on. Use another hot water bottle to cuddle into yourself to help keep your body warm and relaxed at the same time.
- Water! Drink two to three big glasses of water immediately. Some sufferers say this will stop a very early migraine altogether, others do so daily to help prevent them.
- Rest well propped up on pillows. Lying flat tends to make headaches worse.

EMERGENCY HOMEOPATHY

Migraine treatment is usually constitutional (i.e. the homeopath needs to see you in a full consultation and prescribe a remedy not just for the migraine but for your entire system) but in emergencies and at the first sign of an attack, try:

Spigelia 6 if the pain begins at the back of your head then moves to settle above one eye, is made worse by cold and better if you wrap up cosily;

Lycopodium 6 if it's worse on the right, feels as if your temples are being winched together, you're dizzy and when you try to concentrate on anything the pain worsens;

Homeopathic tincture of *feverfew* is also helpful.

HEADACHES (NON-MIGRAINE)

Headaches are so common and can be caused by so many different things, from sinusitis and high blood pressure to working under fluorescent lights, that the medical dictionaries merely define them as ' head pain from a wide variety of causes'. The pain ranges from the mildly annoying to the totally debilitating, but however vicious the headache they are not usually a sign of any serious underlying disorder.

From a physical point of view, headaches are the result of tension or stretching in the muscles of the neck and scalp, tension in the membranes around the brain, or shortage of oxygen (in the same way as being in a stuffy room for hours can give you a cracking head). One of the most common causes of headaches is ice cream. Commonly known as brain freeze it happens after eating ice cold food or drinks says neurologist professor Joseph Hulihan of Temple University Health Center in Philadelphia. Roll on summer.

The most likely causes include:

- hangovers
- dental problems
- allergies
- eyestrain
- fevers
- head or neck or back problems – including poor posture
- anxiety or depression
- stress
- a workplace that's short on fresh air and heavy on artificial lighting
- too much caffeine. Try not to drink more than four cups of tea or coffee a day and less if you seem to be sensitive to it
- low blood sugar levels (when you have not, perhaps, eaten for some time)

- dehydration
- sunstroke – from total prostration to 'a touch of the sun'
- neuralgia and shingles
- the contraceptive pill
- premenstrual syndrome
- the menopause
- head injury
- for some people, powerful negative emotions such as anger
- 'Rebound headaches' after stopping taking prescription medicine, or even mild over-the-counter painkillers is also a possibility.

Note: *headaches that are worse when you wake up, that wake you up at night, or that come on suddenly need to be checked by a doctor, because there are a few more serious underlying causes which need prompt identification and treatment. They include high blood pressure, an aneurysm (ballooning out of a blood vessel) in the brain, inflammation of the arteries in the head or neck, and even, though this is fortunately rare, a brain tumour.*

DIY HEADACHE BUSTER

This is especially useful for office workers, and other people who have to spend much of the day in a sitting position.

Cracking headache? Try the tug

Gently grasp handfuls of your hair right down at the roots. Pull gently and rhythmically six times on each handful, working your way around your head from the back upwards and outwards. This helps because it encourages the release of tension from the tiny muscles underneath your scalp. A tense scalp is an A1 cause of headaches.

The shrug

Sit up straight, forearms resting on lap. Shrug your shoulders up towards your ears as you take a slow breath in. Breathe out deep and slow as you gently let them drop again.

The circle

In the same position circle first one shoulder, three times clockwise, then three times anticlockwise, then the other. This helps release neck muscle tension which is a big contributor to headaches.

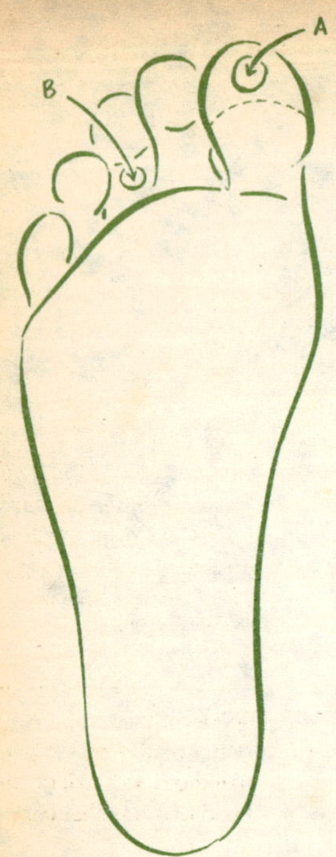

Tackle eyestrain with reflexology. On the soles of both feet, rotate the ball of your thumb on area B firmly for 3 minutes at a time, every hour if necessary. It is important to rest your eyes for at least 30 minutes at a time after doing so. Cracking headache? Soothe it with reflexology. Work the area on the big toe above the dotted line. Use your thumb in a caterpillar movement, to press in a rotating movement for up to 3 minutes at a time, every 30 minutes if necessary. Migraines respond by working area A at the start of an attack.

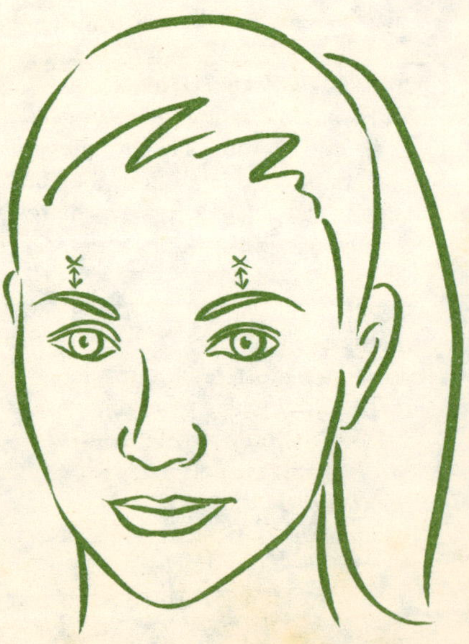

To help calm headaches that hurt around the front of your head, and forehead, find the acupressure point that lies about one thumb's width above the middle of your eyebrow on each side of your head. The Chinese call this the Yangbai point. Apply gentle but firm pressure with your thumbs, smoothing the skin up towards your hairline. This also helps soothe the eyestrain that often goes with this type of headache.

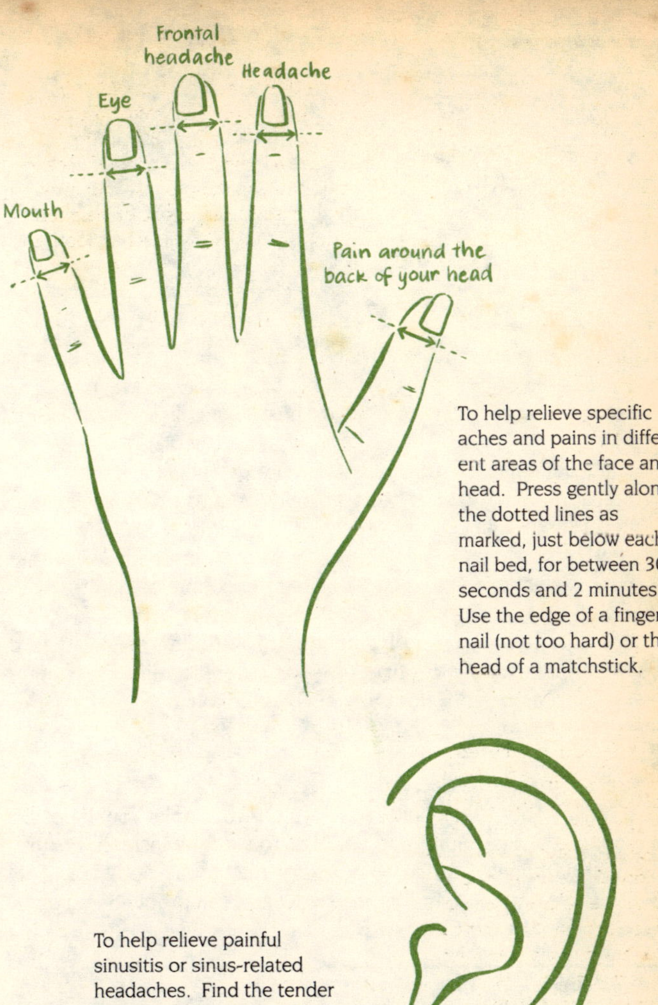

To help relieve specific aches and pains in different areas of the face and head. Press gently along the dotted lines as marked, just below each nail bed, for between 30 seconds and 2 minutes. Use the edge of a fingernail (not too hard) or the head of a matchstick.

To help relieve painful sinusitis or sinus-related headaches. Find the tender spot on your ear as marked and press gently for 2-3 minutes, 2-3 times a day.

The eyebrow rub

Place an index finger on the innermost point of each eyebrow, the part closest to your nose. Rub in small circular movements along the eyebrow, as firmly or as gently as is comfortable, working your way along to the eyebrow outer end. Now do ten circular rubs clockwise on the temple, eleven anticlockwise, and finish the mini-facial massage with ten firm sliding strokes up into your hairline.

Shut your eyes for a minute.

Acupressure power

Hold up your hand (any hand). On the tips of the fingers (as shown in the diagram on p. 95) are the points to work for getting rid of:

- headband-style pain (the finger next along from your index finger)
- headache pulsing in the crown of your head (index finger)
- pain at the back of your head, going down into where it joins the neck (the thumb).

Gently stimulate the corner points in what acupressurists call the Finger's Medial and Lateral nail points for a couple of minutes at a time with the nail edge of a finger from your other hand.

Massage the Hegu 4 point in the soft webbing of your hand between thumb and index finger (see p. 23 for diagram). Press here rotating the area gently, for thirty seconds to a minute, four or five times a day.

Office anti-headache tip

Turn off any fluorescent lights nearby if co-workers let you. If possible bring in a desk lamp, and use that to work by instead. Ensure the bulb is bright – a dim forty watter may look soothing but it doesn't give enough light for close work and can produce eyestrain headaches of its own.

Seeing Green

Colour therapists recommend you stare at something green (not a computer screen, and that piece of cucumber in your lunch time sandwich is way too small). If you can't see anything green about, shut your eyes and visualise a large green circle, lawn, lake or jewel.

Homeopathy

Homeopathy depends on matching the precise type of headache you have (throbbing, nagging, needle-like pain, constant, intermittent etc.) to the right remedy. Possibilities include:

Aconite 30 if your headache arrived suddenly, feels like a tight band around your head and is worse in the cold or draught; *Belladonna* 30 if it's a throbbing pain, worse in hot sun, your face is flushed and pupils a bit dilated;

Byronia 30 if the pain is sharp and stabbing, made worse when you move;

Ignatia 6 if it's like a nail being driven into the side of your head or again, a tight band across your forehead.

HUNG OVER?

- Tomato juice with lots of crushed ice helps replace lost water and salts, accompanied by toast soldiers spread with either honey or Marmite.
- Drink lots of water, as much as you can, for a couple of hours, to help flush your system through and replace lost water.
- White willow extract for the pain. It's similar to aspirin but without the irritating effect on an already upset gut lining.
- Try homeopathy:

  Chamomilla 6 if you are like the textbook 'bear with a sore head' and want everyone to leave you alone;

  Nux Vomica 6 if your head aches as if you have been beaten up, you're feeling dizzy, ratty and dull.

  (for both, try up to six doses at hourly intervals, with plain water to drink in between)
- The herb milk thistle may well boost the body's toxin turnover. When alcohol is absorbed into your bloodstream it has a toxic effect, as well as depleting your mineral and vitamin stores. The familiar result is sickness and a cracking headache. Milk Thistle is thought to help get rid of a hangover because it supports the regeneration of liver cells. Try a convenient supplement called Silymarin Plus (from Larkhall Green Farm), which also has vitamin B in it to encourage the efficient processing of alcohol. It needs to be taken in the six to eight week run up to any serious Party Season, not just the morning after.

IRRITABLE BOWEL SYNDROME (IBS)

IBS is very common in the UK, affects more women than men, and according to the self-help group The IBS Network it affects one in three of us at some time. While it may not be life-threatening it can be both painful and distressing, sending one in ten sufferers to their doctor for help. Sadly, most GPs' understanding of IBS and its effective treatment is still pretty hazy, the treatments they generally offer – usually anti-spasmodic drugs and bulking (fibre) agents – are seldom sufficiently helpful, and there is as yet no definitive cure. Even diagnosis in the first place can be difficult.

So it's not surprising that many people with IBS have got so heartily fed up with this that they are taking the initiative themselves, actively choosing complementary medicine and sensible, practical self-help options to give themselves a good measure of control both over the condition's behaviour, and over their own lives. However, it is important to get medical confirmation that you do have IBS by an understanding, knowledgeable GP or, more likely, by a specialist (a gastroenterologist) with a specific interest in IBS so you can plan your treatment accordingly. It is also vital to be able to rule out the (albeit unlikely) possibility of serious health problems, such as Crohn's disease or ulcerative colitis.

Common IBS symptoms can include:

- sharp abdominal pain and spasm
- diarrhoea (and consequent difficulty in hanging onto a bowel movement), constipation or both
- sharp rectal pain
- uncomfortable tummy bloating
- thunderous, copious wind
- continence problems
- nausea, burping and vomiting.

Note: if you see any blood in your faeces, if you have fever or are losing weight for no apparent reason as well as any of the above symptoms, see your GP right away for a check-up.

IMMEDIATE SELF-HELP MEASURES

The gut has its own rich enteric (intestinal) nervous system. If all its neurons were added together, they would form a mass the size of your brain. That is why herbs and therapies that soothe the nervous system can be so useful for IBS.

- Chamomile tea is carminative (spasm-relieving and wind-reducing), and research shows that it is a good soother and toner for an uptight gut. Make with the dried herb itself (1 heaped teaspoon steeped for three minutes) or with 2-3 gms of powdered chamomile, or 3-4ml of herb tincture. Drink three times daily in between meals.

  Forget the tastefully packed herbal commercial chamomile teas in the supermarket – they are not up to medicinal standard and unlikely to be much use. They also taste pretty insipid. Try a heaped teaspoon of proper dried chamomile flowerheads instead, as apart from anything else they taste much nicer.
- Peppermint, either as a tea or in capsule oil form, helps some but by no means all IBS sufferers. Use one teaspoon of this but brew it up for longer – five minutes. The maximum intake is four cups a day. For the capsule oil form, follow the dosage on the label.
- A tea of fennel seeds, caraway seeds, peppermint and wormwood. Brew one teaspoon of each up together, leave to steep for three to four minutes, drain and drink three times daily. Fennel tea on its own can also be soothing for the tummy and many people reckon it tastes nicer than the mix.
- Homeopathy can be very calming for IBS, and one study at the Royal Hallamshire County Hospital in Winchester in 1991 showed it was just as effective as orthodox medical treatment. A visit to a good homeopath will produce by far

The gut has its own rich enteric (intestinal) nervous system. If all its neurons were added together, they would form a mass the size of your brain

the best results, and they will give you a constitutional treatment instead of just a symptomatic one. However, it may be worth trying these remedies first:

Argentus nit. 6 if you swing between constipation and diarrhoea, with impressive wind to boot, and mucus in the stools;

Colocynth 6 if you have sharp, gripping tummy pains and the only thing that helps them is doubling over, especially if your attacks are linked to anger;

Colchicum can help pain if you are also feeling sick and cannot face the idea of food; German research at Munich's Institut fur Datenanalyse und Versuchplannung in 1976 found that homeopathic treatment with *Asa foetida* was helpful, even in the sort of double blind clinical trials where neither the administering doctors nor the patients knew whether they were getting 'real' medication or not.

- Soothing colours: Do you like the colours orange and green? Colour therapists say these may help as the former is warming and the latter is calming/soothing. They suggest that you wear them over the abdominal area (e.g. warm orange pants, a green skirt) or use a couple of light squares of silk in these vibrant colours tucked into your ordinary knickers or down trouser fronts.
- Stevenage aromatherapist and pathologist Dr Vivienne Lunney suggests trying a gentle tummy and lower back massage with ten drops of grapefruit essential oil in a palmful of plain carrier oil.
- For PMS – IBS: If you get IBS premenstrually, try evening primrose oil – take about 400mg daily in the ten days leading up to your period.

Do you like the colours orange and green? Colour therapists say these may help as the former is warming and the latter is calming/soothing

Other tips from people with IBS include:

- yoga, lying tummy down on a hard floor (takes some practice but reportedly worth it)
- stretching exercises to open the colon
- gentle regular exercise
- natural live yoghurt rich in lactobacillus
- raw chopped garlic added to food (this, however, may actually

irritate some people's IBS)

- low-starch diets
- comprehensive allergy testing
- eating plans high in non-allergenic fibre such as brown rice, oatmeal, vegetables, psyllium husks (a natural bulking agent) and whole wheat.

ALOE VERA – HELP OR JUST HYPE?

On the up side, aloe vera certainly has helped some people with IBS, and it is known to have anti-inflammatory and anti-bacterial properties. On the down side, there are also reports of it actually making IBS worse. There seem to be no studies specifically on its use for IBS available from the producer companies. Aloe vera is expensive, and the IBS network reports that some of its members have been subjected to unwelcome hard-sell approaches from the network marketing distributors of the gel.

LONGER-TERM SELF HELP

Think about doing an Autogenic Training course. This is basically just a fast way to learn deep relaxation (in eight to ten group sessions – whereas with meditation or yoga it usually takes far longer) and has been successfully used to treat IBS, period pains, insomnia and high blood pressure, both within the NHS and privately. It is also effective at shortening childbirth and reducing the pain it can involve.

Costs: approximately £250, or some training may also be available at the London Homeopathic Hospital on the NHS. Contact the British Association for Autogenic Training and Therapy.

A hypnotherapy course. Clinical research at the Wythington Hospital in Manchester in 1994 shows hypnotherapy works well with IBS whether it's gut-directed or general deep relaxation with an affirmation, chosen by you. An affirmation is an instruction your conscious mind gives to your unconscious mind and body, when they are at their most receptive to being programmed. The instruction may be 'I will have no tummy pain tomorrow', 'my guts will be calm', 'my constipation will ease' – whatever you need. A practitioner can show you how to put yourself into a light hypnotic state within a couple of one-to-one sessions, and this is preferable to having a practitioner do it for you, as it can put a good measure of

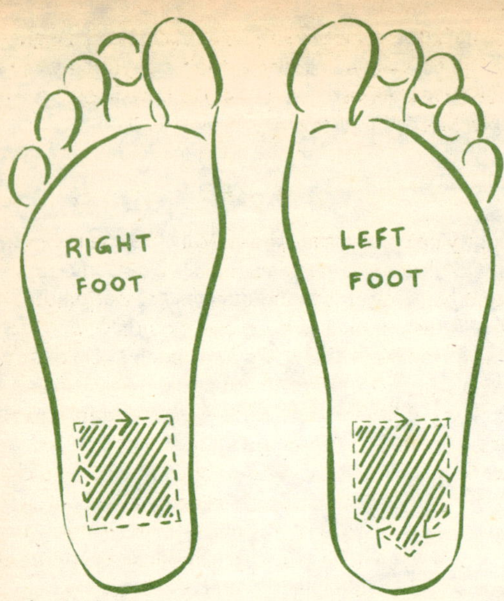

To help relieve IBS press over the shaded areas on the soles of the feet working in the direction of the arrows, as necessary.

control over IBS into your own hands. It is important that your hypnotherapist is professionally qualified (for how to find one via the National Register of Hypnotherapists and Psychotherapists, see p. 144).

Check out what you're eating. Most people with IBS are sensitive to certain foods. See a doctor with an interest in nutrition or a really good nutritionist. Or, as a start, if you suspect certain foods, try making a list of them and leaving one out at a time for a week, seeing if it makes a difference, then introducing it and seeing what happens.

Try a general anti-IBS eating plan if the prospect of turning detective and targeting one suspect food at a time seems just too daunting and finicky. The Women's Nutritional Advisory Service, who have been successfully helping women with the nutritional approach to beating PMS and menopausal symptoms for many years, have devised a 'No More IBS' eating programme, which, after a trial involving 200 people with IBS, they claim helped eighty-seven per cent of participants 'overcome their symptoms completely'. Call them up to ask about it (see p. 144) or have a look at a copy of the book 'No More IBS' (Vermilion, £8.99, 1997).

'SEEING' YOUR PAIN BETTER

Think about trying some visualisation. Many people managing their own long-term chronic pain say that this is a powerful tool in staying on top of pain and just as importantly, something they can do for themselves, which utilises their own body's power to soothe, calm pain and heal itself. If it works for women in childbirth (which it can do very well) it could work for you too.

1. Relax by lying down or semi-reclining comfortably somewhere quiet where you won't be disturbed for at least ten minutes.
2. Breathe deeply (in for eight, hold it for eight, out for eight).
3. See in your mind's eye a warm, healing, golden light growing in your tummy, spreading outwards and becoming slowly brighter.
4. 'See' it soothing, calming, relaxing, caressing your entire abdominal area.
5. Hold that image, and keep reinforcing it, for as long as is comfortable.
6. When you feel you have done enough, don't just open your eyes and leap off the bed. Come back gently and gradually. Let the golden light you built up diminish to a small glow – like the last ember of what was a blazing open fire. Keep that glow with you if you can the rest of the day.
7. Let your breathing return to normal.
8. Then get up.

Do this, if you can, once a day, and also as a practical DIY comforter when the pain is starting to get to you. It can be hard to concentrate on golden glows at first – if you are not used to this sort of thing you may find the image keeps sliding away from you as you remember that you forgot to lock the car up/turn on the supper/send that letter at work. But like relaxation and visualisation classes for labour, the technique gets much easier, and more effective with practise – the more often you do it, the better you get at it, and the more it helps. A lesson or two from a yoga teacher, hypnotherapist or AT trainer (see p. 19) could help you visualise especially powerfully and effectively.

The suggestions in the IBS section may sound so diverse as to have no coherent logic to them, but IBS is a type of gut behaviour not a single clearly defined disease. Like PMS, it is a multisyndrome of many different symptoms, causes and triggers, not a disease with one specific cause and cure. What helps – and there is a great deal which can – depends on what's causing it. Looked at in a positive light, at least this puts a great many options and a high degree of potential control in the hands of the person who has it. The frustrating (and often very tiring) element is tracking down what works best for you personally by a sometimes lengthy process of trial, information seeking and error. But don't give up – somewhere out there, there is something that is going to help you, maybe a little, but maybe a lot.

MOUTH ULCERS

These are small open sores in the form of rounded white, greyish or yellowish spots, with an inflamed red edge. They can turn up anywhere in the soft mucous membrane lining of your mouth, including the insides of the lips, cheeks, or on your tongue. They are painful to touch, sting and may make eating difficult. Causes include ill-fitting braces or dentures, a graze inside the mouth, taking a nip out of your own cheek by mistake while eating, digestive problems, food intolerances and allergies, viral infections, anaemia, gingivitis and being generally tired and run down. Some women find they are more prone to developing ulcers in the ten days before their period begins. They are only very rarely linked with mouth cancer.

ULCER BEATERS

DABBING IT ON

- Tincture of myrrh can clear ulcers up within forty-eight hours. It can sting, but it's usually worth it. Long known for its antibiotic properties, this substance used to be very highly prized (remember the Three Kings' third gift to the infant Christ?). You can make a good mouthwash to help soothe and clear up ulcers. Add ten drops of myrrh tincture to a cup (240ml) of warm, previously boiled water and use twice daily.
- Peppermint tea sipped regularly throughout the day can help to soothe and heal.
- Try mouthwashes preventatively if you know you tend to get ulcers premenstrually – use for a couple of days about a week before your period would usually begin. Two good ones are salty water, or four drops of Bach Flower Rescue Remedy in half a teacup of warm water.

PILLS AND POWDERS

- Be your own homeopath, try:

  Mercurius 6c if your ulcers are mostly on your tongue where they sting and burn, and if you also find you have bad breath and more saliva than is usual for you.

  Arsenicum if your mouth is dry and burning, and the ulcers seem to be soothed by warm water.
- A good vitamin B complex, an all-in-one supplement or a vitamin B and iron tonic such as Floradix can help if you suspect your crop of ulcers may have appeared because you are run down.
- Rinse out your mouth with a warm solution of salt several times a day. Make it with one heaped teaspoon of salt in a glass of boiled, cooled water.

PELVIC INFLAMMATORY DISEASE (PID)

Pelvic inflammatory disease is a catch-all term for any infection or inflammation which has travelled deep into a woman's reproductive system. It's possible to have it for many months, even years, without ever being diagnosed properly – all you know is it hurts to have sex, aches when you walk heavily and that you feel constantly run down.

PID may take the form of a single sharp (acute) attack, or it may grumble on for years as a chronic condition. Short-term symptoms include a temperature, painful sex, vaginal discharge and sometimes vaginal bleeding in between periods. Chronic symptoms include low abdominal pain on one or both sides, infertility or reduced fertility, backache, nausea, constant tiredness and pain when passing water. Possible causes include infections, such as chlamydia, gonorrhoea – there may even be a link with the bacteria causing cystitis. As for how an infection gets 'all the way up there', routes include pelvic surgery, abortion, miscarriage, an IUD and sexual intercourse. PID can be difficult to get rid of once it takes hold, but encouragingly there is a great deal you can do from a self help and DIY complementary therapy point of view to help your body fight off this disorder for good.

If you develop an acute attack, don't ignore it or self treat for any longer than forty-eight hours if matters aren't starting to improve. Take yourself straight off to the nearest big hospital's Special Clinic. Special Clinics, (which also deal with a wide range of sexually transmitted diseases) and major family planning centres if you already belong to one, are the expert treatment and testing centres – this is not a time to go to your GP. The clinic should give you a full spectrum of tests and a hearty cocktail of antibiotics. Take the full course. Go to all follow-up appointments: no one needs chronic PID. It's painful, debilitating, can make sex constantly uncomfortable and may cause permanent infertility too.

IMMEDIATE SELF SOOTHERS

- Self massage, or better still, get your lover or friend to do it: twice daily aromatherapy massage of the lower abdomen and back areas using a combination of rosewood or palmarosa, with lavender (ten drops of each in a palmful of carrier oil such as almond, or at a pinch, soya oil). Former pathologist and aromatherapist Dr Vivienne Lunny from Stevenage explains that these oils are thought to help destroy infectious agents and strengthen the immune system.
- A hot water bottle held cuddled against the pelvic area can help soothe the pain by increasing blood flow and relaxing muscles. Place another one against your lower back too, if this is also aching.
- Take white willow complex (similar to aspirin but without the side effect on the gut).
- Consciously relax. This helps relax the muscles around the pelvic area which have probably tightened up against the pain, and are making it worse. The quickest, easiest way if you have no time for meditation classes is to breathe in for eight, hold it for eight, breathe out for eight. Do this twenty times. Continue if it's calming and helpful. This has a remarkably rapid effect. Just slowing and regulating your breathing slows down your heart and metabolic rate.
- Hurting? After the twenty slow breaths, try some visualisation, literally 'seeing' yourself better in your mind's eye. One of the most effective ways to do this is to imagine a warm golden light spreading over your lower abdomen. Imagine it is soothing as it spreads, comforting and healing. Or imagine golden hands stroking the pain away. Concentrate on keeping the image you have chosen there for a while. Do this as often as you can: every morning before you get up, in the middle of the day if it begins to hurt, and every evening are good times.

LONGER TERM MEASURES

- If you have been given antibiotics, take lactobacillus acidophilus and bifido bacterium supplements (often sold in the same supplement) and pessaries to avoid developing a robust case of thrush on top of everything else.

- Go to bed and rest for several days. PID can be serious. Let your body use its energy for fighting it off, not for work.
- Avoid sex until you are completely better.
- Call the clinic if the pain's not improving within 48 hours.
- Take vitamin C and echinacea supplements for at least three, preferably six, months. Vitamin C is anti-inflammatory, echinacea will boost your immune system's fight against the infection (see pp. 82-3). Medical herbalists such as Mark Evans, past president of the National Institute of Medical Herbalists suggest women with PID take echinacea for several months to stop the problem recurring.
- Stop smoking. It uses up your vitamin C supplies needed for infection fighting, and tobacco causes the smooth fibres of your muscles to contract, which will not help the muscles of your pelvis that are probably already contracted with discomfort.
- Do anything you can to relax and reduce stress. Stress and anxiety cause the pelvic muscles to spasm, again producing more pain. Warm baths to which ten drops of lavender essential oil has been added are both relaxing and analgesic. Relaxation exercises, a bit of meditation and visualisation – it all helps.
- Colour therapists suggest you wear indigo coloured knickers – soft, big ones that come up to the tummy button), trousers, skirts etc. on the area over your abdomen. Some therapists also recommend tucking a square of indigo silk in there instead, as this is regarded as a powerful healing and soothing colour.

> *Short-term symptoms include a temperature, painful sex, vaginal discharge and sometimes bleeding in between periods*

PERIOD PAIN

Nine out of ten women find that they have painful periods (dysmenorrhoea) at least some of the time, a third of these always do. For one in ten it gets so bad that they cannot even get into work for at least a day, according to research by the University of California in 1996. It's thought that women with bad period pain may have extra-powerful womb contractions to thank for this, either because they are producing more of the hormone-like substances prostaglandins, which cause uterus contractions, or because they are just more sensitive to ordinary amounts.

Stress, anxiety and overwork are other major period-pain worseners

Varying from a sharp cramping sensation around the lower abdomen to a dull dragging ache there or in your lower back, the feeling can also spread down the upper insides of your thighs. Some women find it is severe enough to make them feel physically sick. Common causes include fibroids, endometriosis, a pelvic infection (suspect this especially if you have an intra-uterine device (IUD) – and IUDs can be associated with heavier, more painful periods anyway), coming off the Pill, and plain getting older as menstrual patterns do start changing past the age of thirty-five. Stress, anxiety and overwork are other major period-pain worseners. Always see your GP if periods have become suddenly more painful, or heavier.

Painful periods might clear up after you've had your first baby. But up to a third of women find they actually get worse – and heavier – as if labour has made the womb more reactive to prostaglandins and more efficient at contracting powerfully (one possible reason why second/subsequent labours are blessedly faster than first time ones).

THE ANTI-PERIOD PAIN PLAN

1. *Lie down comfortably* on your side with a hot water bottle on your lower back/lower tummy, and a squashy pillow between your knees, supporting the abdomen.

or

Lie on your back, with your head and shoulders well supported, and your knees bent with a pillow to raise them up, hot water bottle at the ready.

Do either of these for twenty to thirty minutes.

Then take:

2. A *warm bath*. Add ten drops of lavender essential oil for its pain-relieving properties. Used by nurses at Oxford's John Radcliffe hospital for women in labour (a very similar pain for similar reasons – but more so) with a sixty per cent success rate for relieving labour discomfort.
3. *The herb white willow complex*. If you want an easy to take natural pain killer in tincture or pill form try white willow (the tree from which modern aspirin was developed), 1-2ml every four hours. Aspirin is very useful for many types of pain including period cramps, but some people don't like using it because it can irritate the lining of the stomach.
4. *An anti-period pain herbal drink*. Make a comforting, pain-soothing tea with one heaped teaspoon of dried herb in a cup of boiling water, leaving it to steep for four minutes and drink without milk or sugar – use a little honey if it improves the taste instead. The appropriately named cramp bark is a good muscle relaxant. If the problem is relatively mild and annoying rather than crippling, take chamomile tea with a little ginger and honey added to make it taste nicer. Black cohosh is a traditional remedy for general muscle spasm as well as menstrual cramp.
5. *Try gentle* DIY *homeopathic remedies* every hour, up to ten doses worth, as soon as the period pain begins, suggests homeopathic GP Dr Andrew Lockie:

   Belladonna 6 if the pain is worse before the blood flow even begins, and it's an aching dragging feeling, you don't feel any better for lying down and when the flow begins it's a bright red colour.

   Pulsatilla 30 if you feel miserably weepy and sick, but the period flow itself is light.

   Magnesia phos. 30 if heat and firm pressure help (perhaps a hot water bottle cuddled firmly against the area), if movement helps, and if the pain arrives in spasms.

   Sepia 30 (one dose to be taken three times a day just before periods begin or on the first day) if the pain is dull, powerful, dragging and the flow is very heavy with large, gelly-like clots.

   Chamomilla 30 if you are irritable and restless and the pains are cramp-like and severe.

   One German trial carried out in 1993 on 133 women with

painful periods, using a general constitutional homeopathic remedy containing belladonna, sulfuricum, colcocynthis and dioscorea found that in eighty-five per cent of cases, results were either 'good' or 'very good'.

Note: the best results are obtained if you can get to see a homeopath who will prescribe something which will suit you and your medical history very specifically.

6. *Try gentle movement*:

- Rest down on your knees, stretch out your neck and arms so that your elbows are on the floor in front of you, head between your arms in the yoga Cat Stretch position. Stay there for as long as is comfortable.
- Gentle exercise, such as swimming or walking, especially in the few days before your period is due to begin.

PAIN-BUSTING TIP

Take painkillers, whether natural or pharmaceutical drugs, before it really starts hurting you. Preferably when you get the first vicious warning signs. If you wait till it's really hurting the nerve endings will be in a more reactive state, and will respond powerfully to even weak pain signals. Dentists' patients are often asked to take painkillers before they have a nasty filling rather than after for the same reason.

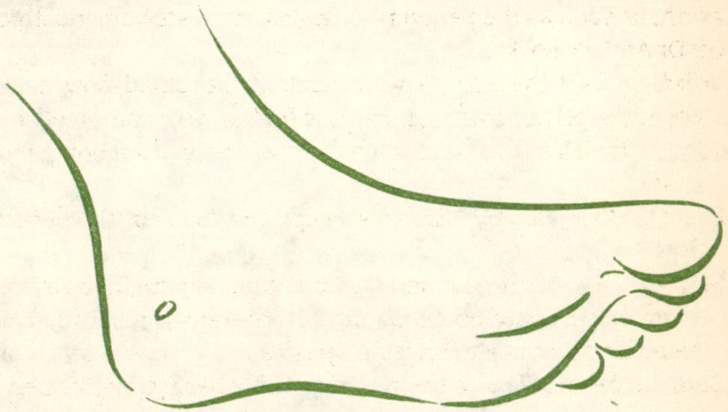

The area relating to your uterus (womb) is the small circle. To soothe period pain using reflexology press a thumb's width around this area gently but firmly for 3 minutes at a time over a period of 20 minutes until the pain recedes.

PRESS HERE FOR PAIN RELIEF
There is a very useful pressure point which acupuncturists call Shousanli that can help soothe most types of abdominal pain. To find it place your index finger in the crease of your elbow, slide it down a couple of inches on the outside of the arm. Feel around gently until you find the area that's especially sensitive and rotate the ball of your thumb there gently for four or five minutes. Have a twenty minute break and repeat. Or try the L 4 Hegu point (see diagram p. 23) which is more of a general point for pain.

PROSTATITIS

This is inflammation of the prostate, an unobtrusive little accessory sex gland that lies at the base of a man's bladder. A prostate is about the size of the average walnut and curls around the urethra, the tube that carries urine from the bladder down into the penis. Prostate problems are usually associated with older men (eg an enlarged prostate can make peeing difficult) but prostatitis affects younger men in their twenties, thirties and forties, and tends to be painful from the start. It has been nicknamed the Silent Scream because it can be so very uncomfortable, and men can have it for some time without knowing what is wrong. Prostatitis also tends to be hard to diagnose, and to treat.

Regarded as being the male equivalent of women's PID (Pelvic Inflammatory Disease see p. 106) it can cause a very wide range of painful symptoms. For the long term, grumbling variety, these include:

- lower-back pain
- painful sex and urination
- pain in the perineum area between anus and scrotum
- painful ejaculation

- premature ejaculation
- pain in the lower abdomen, testes, groin, inner thighs and penis
- a frustratingly slow, trickling urine flow.

Causes are as varied as the symptoms, but may include:

- Infection. Urologists are currently putting their money on chlamydia.
- Stress and worry (prostatitis is most often seen in the high-achieving Type A personality men). The reason is that according to Julian Shar, consultant urologist at London's Institute of Urology, anxiety can contribute to pelvic floor muscle spasms.

KEEP IT COMING

Not ejaculating that often can cause a build up of fluids in the prostate gland which can produce local irritation and may be enough to start off inflammation in the area. So if you are into Tantric sex, wherein the man only rarely ejaculates, watch it.

SELF HELP

- Stay off anything that worsens or triggers attacks. The usual suspects are caffeine (in tea, coffee and cola drinks), spicy foods and alcohol – try low/no-alcohol lagers or beers. They taste a lot better if properly chilled.
- Cut down or stop smoking. The nicotine in tobacco causes the smooth fibres of the muscles to contract, making any existing prostate pain worse.
- If you are the slightest bit constipated, eat at least four to five portions of fresh fruit and drink at least 1½–2 litres of water daily, as straining to empty the bowels puts extra pressure on a sore prostate and can make any inflammation worse.
- Take anti-oxidant vitamins A, C and E as they can help reduce inflammation.
- Consider a zinc supplement. Cases of prostatitis have often been linked to not enough zinc in the prostate fluid. As zinc competes with copper for absorption by the body, most nutritionally orientated doctors are also likely to suggest

Cases of prostatitis have often been linked to not enough zinc in the prostate fluid taking 2-3mg of copper daily as well.

- For a sudden acute attack, the following homeopathic remedies may be useful – keep them in the medicine cabinet if you are prone to prostatitis bouts. Take every two hours for up to ten doses.

  Thuja 6c if you can feel a burning at the neck of your bladder and want to pass water a lot.

  Sabal 6 if intercourse is painful and you cannot ejaculate.

  Pulsatilla 6 if you keep needing to pass water and find you cannot seem to wait to do so, if lying on your back makes it all feel worse, and if there is some thick yellow discharge from your penis.

  If symptoms do not subside within 24 hours, see your GP.

  However, homeopaths strongly advise that prostatitis needs constitutional treatment, i.e. one that is customised for you personally following a long consultation and medical history taking. So for best results, book yourself an appointment (see p. 143).

HERBS FROM YOUR UROLOGIST

A non-drug, natural medicine called Cernilton, which is a mix of pollens from certain plants growing in southern Sweden, often succeeds where all else has failed. Trials at Cardiff's University of Wales, the Royal Infirmary in Glasgow and Germany's Georg-August University at Gottingen found about seventy per cent of men with hard-to-shift prostatitis did well with this. You need to take it for at least three months to see any results. A specialist (urologist) can prescribe this for you, as, if you can convince them, can your GP. If they think this sounds a bit fringe and are not keen, try telling them (truthfully) that it's so respectable that it's registered as a pharmaceutical in Austria, Switzerland, Japan, Korea, Germany, Argentina, Spain and Greece.

JOCK TIP

If you play sport, run or jog, have a really good pee before each session or game. Vigorous exercise on a full or partially full bladder is a risk factor for prostatitis, possibly because the shaking up and down could encourage prostate fluid to trigger irritation, which may go on to become full-scale inflammation, in the delicate channels inside the gland itself.

REPETITIVE STRAIN INJURY (RSI)

RSI is a blanket term for a wide range of over-use injuries, and because it doesn't have a clear medical definition it gets called many different things. One doctor will say you have tenosynivitis, another mutters 'tendinitis' or 'carpal tunnel syndrome'. You may be told it's 'actually, occupational over-use upper limb disorder', 'regional pain disorder', 'cumulative trauma disorder' or 'occupational over-use syndrome'.

But do you have a weakness in the muscles/joints of your arms, hands or fingers? Tingling in the fingers, swelling, pain that persists there even when you are not doing anything? Do your fingers make flicking movements without being asked to? These are all classic RSI symptoms. And your job is often a dead give away. If you have a job where you have to make repetitive arm or hand movements all day while sitting/standing still (a journalist typing, violinist, pizza-cutter, a typist, a switchboard operator, supermarket check-out clerk, computer programmer) combined with an uncomfortable chair, desk, or a poorly aligned work tools set up – you are at risk. If your job is also stressful, you are especially so.

SEX AND VIOLINS

If you are a female string player – whether it's Mozart for the London Philharmonic, or belting Irish folk-rock down the Shamrock and Ferret on a Saturday night – you are twice as likely as a male fiddler to develop RSI.

RSI is traditionally hard to treat, and is often confused with, and treated as, arthritis, which is no help at all. However, like all over-use injuries it gets better fastest and most completely if you catch it early rather than trying to soldier on at work until things become unbearable. Basically, treatment consists of:

- stopping whatever it was that you were doing to cause it
- painkillers

- steroid injections and anti-inflammatory drugs
- physical therapy. Options include physiotherapy, water therapy, the Alexander technique, advice and treatment from an osteopath or chiropractor, who can look at how you work and suggest some ergonomically-friendly improvements (desk height, seating/standing position, use of hands-free equipment).

RSI SELF HELP

Depending on which bits are affected: the following are all well worth trying while you are waiting for medical treatment to work, or for an appointment with an osteopath/chiropractor:

- Stop work temporarily and rest. A lot easier said than done, but if you struggle on you may cause so much damage that you won't be able to do your job ever again.
- Take the herb white willow: it's similar to aspirin but without the side effects on your gut.
- Medical aromatherapist Dr Vivienne Lunney, in Stevenage, suggests a soothing, anti-inflammatory aromatherapy oil mixture of two drops of lavender, two of rosemary and two of juniper. Add to a palmful of plain carrier oil, such as safflower, sunflower or almond, and rub in to the affected area.
- A DIY massage for your own hands or neck and shoulders (two of the most common RSI hot spots) is three drops of Roman Chamomile essential oil mixed with a palmful of carrier oil (sunflower cooking oil is fine at a pinch). Research suggests that it may have anti-inflammatory and painkilling properties.
- Certain nutritional supplements may be good alternatives to painkilling drugs. D-phenylalanine and L-tryptophan (not available at the moment over the counter but may be again soon) are two of these (see p. 153). The latter even helps after tooth extraction and root canal work (see p. 153).
- Rub a little wintergreen oil onto the sore areas – it contains the same stuff as aspirin, salicylate.
- A supplement of vitamin B6 may help, suggests neurologist Dr

> *If you are a coffee addict, switch to tea until your* RSI *is better, or try hot drinks like* Bovril, *or powdered soups*

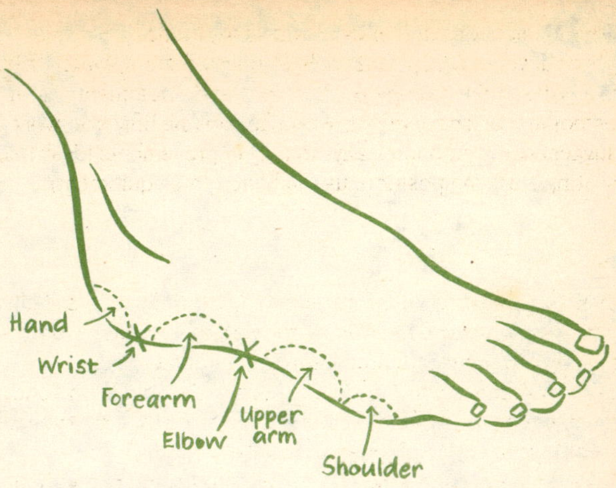

To help relieve RSI using reflexology. Press gently but firmly on the relevant area, working it for approximately 3 minutes, 5 times a day.

Shreyas Patel, medical director of the Pain and Stress Reduction Program at the Marino Center for Progressive Health in Boston.

- Short term: if it's a wrist problem try a wrist splint to support and relax the area.
- Long term: check out your workplace ergonomics (a good osteopath, or even a retail outlet such as the Back Shop, could advise).
- Coffee can increase the pain. Switch your cuppa. If you are a coffee addict, switch to tea until your RSI is better, or try hot drinks like Bovril, or powdered soups. Research (see p. 153) shows that instant coffee blocks up the opiate receptors in rats' brains, which makes them more sensitive to all types of pain. If it happened to them, it could happen to you...

SHINGLES, HERPES AND COLD SORES

Shingles is a painful condition which can persist for months, sometimes years, and be completely debilitating. It's caused by the same virus that produces chicken-pox, attacking and inflaming a nerve, or nerve cell bodies. It shows itself as a blistered rash, usually on the tummy or chest, that looks like a girdle stretching half way around the body. You can also sometimes get it on your face. In Britain, a quarter of a million people develop shingles each year.

This painful rash only ever develops in people who have had chicken-pox at some point, because when your body defeats this (usually) childhood disease, it retreats to the junction box of nerves at the base of the spine, and here it skulks until something triggers it off again, this time in the form of shingles. That something may be becoming run down or unwell, no one is sure, and there are probably multiple different trip-switches.

Shingles is not catching. Its first warning signs are an itching, tingling and burning under the skin; pain, which can be vicious, stabbing and tends to track the pathway of the infected nerve; feeling tired; even a slight temperature. It is now thought to be good medical practice to treat the disease with a powerful anti-viral agent immediately it shows itself, to help avoid a complication called Post Herpetic Neuralgia (see below). So if you are getting the above symptoms, go and see your GP right away and you may head off, or at least damp down, the force of the attack.

Next come fluid-filled blisters which pop up along the nerve route. They burst, weep and turn into sores, then slowly get better over a time span of two to five weeks. The skin then crusts over and heals, possibly leaving behind a bit of sensitivity or nerve ache, as it's called. Even this should disappear soon afterwards (within the month).

If it doesn't, go and see your GP right away as you may have developed a condition called Post Herpetic Neuralgia (PHN) though prompt medication can help avoid PHN altogether. This can last for months, even years. The pain it causes varies from mildly annoying to intense. It can also cause your skin to become so sensitive that for some it is painful even to have light clothing touching the area.

Don't panic if you do have PHN. It can be severe and hard to deal with, but with good treatment nine out of ten people recover from it completely, so long as they get medical help promptly. 'Promptly' was originally defined as being 'within three months'. However according to Boston neurologist and pain specialist Dr Shreyas Patel, the time frame is now 'the sooner the better'. Do not wait a week or two to see if it improves on its own because the longer you leave it, the further this reduces your chances of getting better.

Treatments include very small doses of the more old-fashioned anti-depressants like Amitriptyline, which work rather better for PHN than they ever did for depression. Traditional painkillers tend not to be much use. If the treatments do not help within about four weeks, insist on a referral to a specialist Pain Clinic. There are about 200 of these centres in the UK.

In Britain, a quarter of a million people develop shingles each year

SELF HELP FOR PHN

Different tactics seem to help different people, but here are some of the DIY pain-relieving techniques that former PHN sufferers say helped them:

- Ice packs (see p. 120).
- If clothing touching the skin hurts, try wrapping clingfilm over the area. There is also a medical plastic spray called Opsite (available on prescription from your GP).
- Some people who have PHN say pressing really firmly on the area helps. If it does for you, use a broad sash of light cotton material, bandolier or cummerbund style, to hold a pad of cotton or lint against the area that is hurting.
- TENS machines. Though they are not natural in that they are made of metal and plastic and run on electricity, they utilise the gate theory of pain-signal interruption and trigger the body's natural endorphins (painkillers).
- Capsaicin cream, made from red hot peppers. This destroys the receptors for the neurotransmitter substance P so you feel the pain/discomfort far less.

BEATING SHINGLES PAIN

- Soothe the rash with ice cubes wrapped in a plastic bag, covered by a soft t-shirt or flannel. A pack of frozen peas or sweetcorn (bash out the lumps first) helps too. Keep refreezing your personal shingles pack as necessary. Don't cook with its contents later – you don't need food poisoning on top of everything else.
- Dab neat tea tree or lavender oil on the rash using a cotton bud. If your skin is really sensitive, use the gentler Roman chamomile instead, or blend it with a little plain base cream (such as aqueous cream from the pharmacist) or petroleum gel (like Vaseline) first.
- If your shingles attack is just beginning, homeopaths say it can often be cut short. The following may be helpful (Dr Andrew Lockie suggests as a general guide taking a remedy every 2 hours for up to 10 doses while waiting to see your GP). For further information see his book A *Family Guide to Homeopathy* and also contact a professional homeopath for a personal consultation.

  Rhus tox 6c if your skin is red, blistered and itchy and if warmth and moving helps.

  Ranunculus 6c if you have nerve pains, itching too, and if even small movements/light touches make it all worse.

  Apis 6c if your skin is burning and stinging.

  Arsenicum if the pains burn, are worse between midnight and 2am, and if more blisters are coming up and merging together.

  Mezereum if the pain is really severe, your skin itches, burns and the blisters form into brownish scabs, and if the person is middle aged or elderly.

  Rhus tox may help if the skin is blistered, itchy and red, if the scalp is affected too, if warmth and moving about help, or if the person is young.
- If the rash has gone but the *après* shingles pain just won't quit, try taking a good vitamin B complex with some L-lysine (an amino acid available in health food shops) which is said to shorten some attacks. Herpes simplex (cold sores) is another form of the same virus that causes shingles – take 1000-3000mgs vitamin C daily to boost the immune system.
- *Fire Away*. Capsaicin cream, made from the fiery seeds of hot chilli peppers, can help because it destroys the nerve endings which react to a neurotransmitter called Substance P.

- Colour therapists say that the colour indigo purple helps give inner calmness and is often used to treat neurological disorders, so try wearing clothing in this shade over the area that's affected (e.g. a t-shirt worn under other clothes that covers your abdomen if that is where the shingles rash has broken out). According to therapist Janet James, lecturing at The Herpes Viruses Association's 'Alternative Therapies Day', food in the right colours can also help. Anyone keen on aubergines and fresh purple figs? Yellow is another option colour therapists may use by shining yellow light on the area.

If clothing touching the skin hurts, try wrapping clingfilm over the area

HERPES

Herpes is a virus infection, and it is so common that nine out of every ten of us have had it at some point and carry it, with or without recurring symptoms. The UK is having something of an epidemic at the moment with 27,500 cases of genital herpes alone in 1997, an all time high, so if you have it you are certainly not alone.

It can take several different forms, including shingles, chickenpox and herpes simplex. The latter's available to all comers in two different varieties;

Type 1, which usually produces cold sores around your mouth, nose, and occasionally eyes, genitals and anus.

Type 2 which usually causes sores on the genitals, but just to confuse everyone can also sometimes do so around the mouth.

Due to lack of space, this small section is going to look at what you can do yourself to help soothe the discomfort of genital, and

Fire Away. Capsaicin cream, made from the fiery seeds of hot chilli peppers, can help because it destroys the nerve endings which react to a neurotransmitter called Substance P

mouth herpes sores, which are the two most common sites.

Warning signs of herpes include a tingling or itching feeling where a sore is about to appear, and some people also say they have a nerve ache around the area too. Blister(s) then pop up on dry skin such as the face; ulcers (often extremely sore) form on wet skin, such as the delicate membranes lining a woman's labia. These burst after twenty-four to forty-eight hours leaving small, red, painful ulcers which crust over if they are on dry skin, and get better within three to ten days. You might also feel generally run down, flu-y and have swollen glands in your groin. The best place to go right away if you develop a genital sore like this is your local hospital's GU Dept or special clinic. They will diagnose and treat you fast, efficiently and in total confidence. Take cold sores to your GP, if they do not respond to treatment bought from the pharmacist or self help.

The best news about herpes is:

- If you do have an attack, there is a forty:sixty chance you'll never, ever have another one.
- Any repeat performances can be worked around very effectively, especially important if the sores are around the genitals and you fear for your sex life.
- There are a lot of simple DIY measures which can help enormously with any pain or discomfort it is causing you.

SELF HELP

- Wrap up some frozen peas/sweetcorn/ice cubes in a clean soft cloth and hold them against the area.
- Frozen sandwich soothers – create special thin, flexible ice-packs which are more comfortable and effective than big, lumpy ones. Wet several men's cotton handkerchiefs in water and put them in between alternate layers of polythene, sandwich-style (a cut up supermarket carrier is fine) and place in the freezer. Peel off each one as you need it, fold or roll it into the shape you need and lay against the sore area. As the cooling effect of one frozen hankie wears off, refold it so that another iced area lies comfortingly against the sore.

Note: do not refreeze handkerchiefs. After use wash in the hot cycle of the washing machine. Do not attempt to cook and eat the thawed out veg in case you get food poisoning on top of everything else.

- Dab on witch hazel when you don't have an ice pack clamped to the area. It helps the sores to dry out.
- Bathe the sore areas in salt solution to encourage healing and reduce soreness. Use one tablespoon of salt dissolved in a pint of warm water.
- For genital sores, add a huge handful of salt to your bath water and soak.
- *Peeing comfortably.* If it stings and burns when you pass water, keep a bottle of water by the loo and pour it over your genitals as you pee. Carry a small plastic one around in your bag/briefcase/coat pocket to fill and pour with in loos outside your home. Or pee in a warm bath or under a gentle shower with the water directed at the right place, or into a bidet with the fountain going gently (disinfect well afterwards).
- Try the natural painkiller white willow. It's similar to aspirin, but without the side effects on the gut (available from health shops, or mail order companies such as FSC, see pp. 144-5)
- Slices of cucumber that's been kept in the fridge (or had a ten minute chill-boost in the freezer) are good cold/genital sore soothers.

BE YOUR OWN HOMEOPATH

If you cannot get to the GU clinic or the GP for a few days, try the following as holding measures – they may also help heal the herpes anyway. Take the relevant remedy four times a day for up to two weeks. A visit to the homeopath for a constitutional treatment (personalised for your entire system) to help prevent more attacks is a very good idea.

Rhus tox 6c if your genitals really itch and burn, and you are generally restless.

Natrum mur. 6c if the genital skin is dry, the sores puffy and hot with 'pearl like' fluid blisters.

Capiscum 6c if the skin is cracked, red and painful with a red itchy rash.

SPEED UP HEALING BY:

- Taking 1000-3000mgs vitamin C daily; echinacea tincture/tablets, or zinc supplements (see pp.82-3) to boost your immune system and shorten the herpes attack.
- If it's genital herpes, keep the area cool, wear cotton/silk under-

pants, avoid tight fitting trousers, wear stockings or gussetless tights rather than ordinary tights.

> ***Peeing comfortably:* If it stings and burns when you pass water, keep a bottle of water by the loo and pour it over your genitals as you pee**

- Elagen, a supplement made from the ES plant – short for Eleutherococcus senticosus – with alleged immune-boosting properties might be worth a try. One hundred and eight members of the Herpes Viruses Association took part in a double blind placebo controlled trial of it – and the results were that people taking ES had shorter, fewer and less severe outbreaks. Mail order details from the HVA (see p. 143).
- Take an amino acid (available from health shops) called Lysine. About 500-1000mg a day is the usual dose.
- Take garlic: it's a good general anti-bacterial/anti-viral agent (see p. 153). Try the deodorised but medical-standard tablets such as Kwai's (from health shops).
- Research suggests (see p. 153) that a diet high in lysine and low in arginine can help prevent herpes coming back. High-lysine foods include vegetables, legumes, fish, turkey and chicken. High-arginine foods include chocolate, peanuts, and seeds.
- Orange for the sexual organs, indigo for ulcers say colour therapists. If you have genital herpes, why not try livening up your knicker collection with these colours? Cold sores around the mouth? How about plenty of tangerines (mind the juice on the sore) carrots, purple grapes, aubergines and purple figs to eat?

CHEATING LOVERS

If your lover suddenly develops a herpes sore somewhere personal, do not immediately assume they must have been putting it about on the quiet. Chances are, they haven't. An original herpes infection really can lie dormant for months, even years, then suddenly flare up again. But beware – the other rumours are true. Cold sores are so infectious that you can catch them from kissing someone who is just starting one, even though it barely shows.

COLD SORES

These are painful, itchy little blisters which can develop on the face, usually around the nose and mouth. There may be just one, there may be a crop of them. When the raised blister bursts, the resulting fluid forms a golden crust. They are caused by the highly infectious herpes simplex virus Type 1, which most adults carry, and are more likely to affect you if you are very tired and run down, or have had a recent illness that has depleted your immune system.

Many people have one episode of cold sores but never get another, others may find the sores have a depressing tendency to break out regularly each time they become very tired, ill, stressed or run down. Strong sunlight can be another trigger, though the sores are the last thing you need on a beach or skiing holiday.

COLD SORE SOOTHERS

- Dab a single drop of tea tree or bergamot oil on the area, using a cotton bud.
- Gently rubbing in vitamin E oil to the area can aid healing. Rubbing in garlic oil (break open a garlic oil capsule) can have the same effect.
- Homeopathic help:

  Rhus tox 6c if you have ulcers around the corners of your mouth and your chin is also affected.

  Natrum mur. 6c if the problem's puffy little sores with 'pearl-like' blisters in their centres, accompanied by a dry mouth and a crack in your lower lip.

(Dr Andrew Lockie suggests taking these four times a day for up to five days.)

HOW TO SEE OFF A COLD SORE

To help get rid of the infection, nutritionists often suggest vitamin A, E and zinc supplements, taking garlic internally (one raw clove a day) or taking echinacea, to boost the immune system, (see pp. 82-3) available both as a loose dried herb and also in easier-to-take tablet form.

As a general immune system stimulant, try taking the capsules for three months – 900mg a day. If you have the liquid form (such as the one from FSC's Herbcraft range) take just 3-4ml three times a day. The American Indians used echinacea for snake bites and wounds but when white American doctors first started using it in 1887 they were touting it as a cure-all for anything from VD to the common cold.

SORE THROAT

A sore throat is a blanket term for inflammation/infection of the tonsils, adenoids, larynx, pharynx or vocal cords. It may be all over the back of the mouth, throat and upper breathing tube, or more localised, having zoned in on just the tonsils, for instance. It is also one of the most common physical complaints there is and is described in the medical dictionaries as 'painful throat irritation', though it can vary from a vaguely annoying furry, dry, mildly itchy feeling in the back of the throat to a sensation not unlike swallowing ground glass.

The irritation caused by infection and/or inflammation of the mucous membranes lining the throat can be the fault of a viral or a bacterial infection – colds are the most common culprits – exposure to unfriendly chemicals, cold or very hot, drying air (especially if it's polluted as well – Delhi Throat is almost as famous as Delhi Belly). If a sore throat doesn't start improving a bit within two days for a child, or three days for an adult despite all your self help measures, go to your GP.

HOW TO SOOTHE A THROAT FAST

The following can all be very helpful:

- *Gargling* – with warm salt water is better than nothing at a pinch, but you'll get far better results (soothing and anaesthetic) with a DIY herbal infusion of strong red sage, or goldenseal tea. Take one to two teaspoons of dried red sage or goldenseal (fresh if you've got it but most people haven't) – steep the herbs in a cup of boiling water for three to six minutes, depending on how sore your throat is, strain and gargle three or four times with the mixture for as long as you can. Or do it the easy way: take it as a few drops of tincture, in water.

Gargle four times a day, and if you wake with a desert throat at night, gargle at night too. Do not swallow it – though it's unlikely you'd be tempted to as it tastes vile. You may want to rinse your tongue afterwards as the taste can be strong and bitter, but it has a blessedly anaesthetising effect on a painful throat, and also helps fight infection. Goldenseal helps by soothing the irritated mucous membranes in the throat. The rest of the infusion will keep in the fridge for up to twenty-four hours.

- *Take vitamin C.* At the first sniff of a cold or rasp of a sore throat take 1000mgs and repeat 3-4 times a day until the symptoms subside, reducing the dosage and increasing the time intervals over the next two days. If you start to develop mild diarrhoea, decrease the dose. Britain's Common Cold Unit may not have been convinced by Vitamin C but there are many other separate pieces of good clinical research that suggest it works well (see p. 153 for a review of some of them).

Wear a blue silk scarf round your throat area

- Take the herb echinacea (available in tablet and tincture form) which also protects and boosts the immune system, and though this is not directly related to soothing the pain of an existing sore throat, it will certainly help stop you getting the next one.
- Keep drinking plenty of chilled, or hot, plain fluids throughout the day and evening – ice-cold diluted juice, steaming herbal or milk-less green teas sweetened with honey (also soothing for the throat). If a small child or baby has a miserably sore throat but doesn't want to drink much, make some DIY lollies in the freezer compartment using their own favourite fruit juice flavour. Very diluted Ribena, orange or apple juice are favourites, and let them suck on the lollies for as long as, and as often as, they want.
- Don't smoke at all – not while your throat hurts or is struggling to get better, even if you have a robust twenty-a-day habit. Chew Nicorette gum or put a nicotine patch on from the pharmacist

instead, even if it's just for the next three or four days (a week if you can possibly manage it) to stave off the raging withdrawal symptoms. Stay out of smoky atmospheres and do not let anyone light up near you either.

- Homeopathy can help greatly if you are able to use the right remedy, but go and see a homeopath for best results. The remedy depends on the exact type of sore throat you have. Recognise any of the following?

Dulcamara 6c if your pain and soreness are all on the right, you feel like you have a lump in your throat, you're thirsty but not hungry, your lips are dry and your glands are swollen.

Gelsenium 6c if it hurts when you swallow (even if you're drinking) you feel hot, tired, weak and wobbly and there's a nasty taste in your mouth.

Aconite 30*c* if your sore throat came on suddenly, if it's red, feels burning and tight, your tonsils are swollen, you are really thirsty and cold winds make it worse.

German research in 1976 with doctors in several cities taking

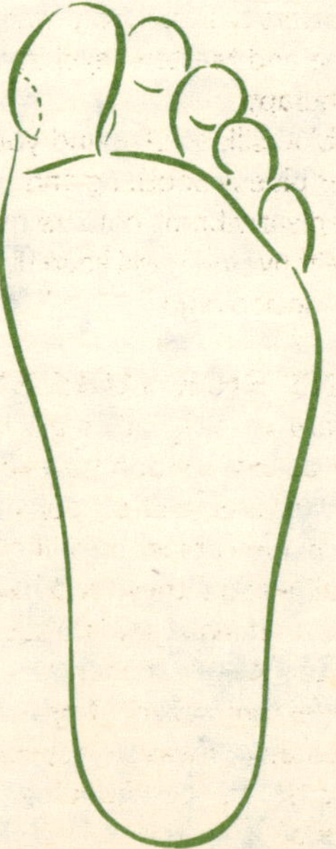

To help soothe a sore throat, gently work the area marked with the ball of your thumb in a circular motion for 3 minutes, 5 times a day. If your sore throat is really acute, do this every half hour.

part (Stuttgart, Bremen, Leipzig) also found *Phytolacca* useful. (Dr Andrew Lockie suggests four times a day for up to seven days.)

A great throat-soothing homeopathic gargle is *Hypericum and Calendula*: five drops each of the mother tincture (available from mail-order homeopathic pharmacies – see pp. 144-5, these can be with you in twenty-four hours) in half a pint of cooled, boiled water. Gargle every four hours in the day, and if you wake at night when the throat is often at its sorest.

- *Aroma-soothe your throat*. Mix five drops each of lavender and tea tree essential oils into a palmful of plain carrier (almond oil is best, sunflower cooking oil will do at a pinch). Rub the lotion gently onto
  - your neck glands,
  - the glands under your arms,
  - glands in the fold of your groin.
  - Rub the remaining oil well into your palms, and
  - the arches of your feet where the blood supply is rich.

  These two oils have anti-infective qualities, according to recent research by biochemist Dr Lis-Balchin, senior lecturer at South Bank University in London, where she has pioneered a new unit at degree and Masters level in the science of Essential Oils and Aromatherapy
- Wear a blue silk scarf round your throat area. Colour therapists say clear blue is soothing and healing. Silk is light and it can be dyed in clear vibrant colours more effectively than, say, cotton; it's non-itchy, and it will keep the area warm – but not too hot, as a woolly scarf would.

PREVENT SICK TUBE SYNDROME

You've heard of sick building syndrome. Now there's sick tube syndrome, as any London traveller can tell you. Wherever fresh air ventilation is poor and air goes around and around any system (including plane cabins) so will germs. If there is air conditioning and central heating, these too have a drying effect on the mucous membranes and make sore throats as well as full blown colds more likely, and can double the length of any infection you already have. During winter if you are cold-prone, take 1000mgs of vitamin C daily as a preventative measure especially if you work in a large office building with air conditioning or commute on the London Underground.

THRUSH

Thrush is not actually an infection, though it sure feels like one. It's an overgrowth of the tiny yeast (fungal) organism Candida Albicans. Probably the most painful place to have it is around the vagina and vulva, though thrush infection of the nipples is not unusual for breast feeding women, and can be miserably sore and itchy (see p. 46-7).

The warning signs of vaginal thrush include a thick pale discharge like curd cheese; a sore, red, itchy vulval area which may sting mercilessly when you pee; painful sex and sometimes a reddish rash extending to the anus, or the inner thighs. Causes include:

- that recent course of antibiotics you finished
- immuno-supressive drugs
- a tired or weakened immune system (perhaps after a prolonged illness or severe stress)
- hormonal change – it's more common in the last week of your menstrual cycle, and when you are pregnant.

GIVING THRUSH THE BRUSH-OFF

SIT IT OUT

- Bathing your vulva in strong, cooled chamomile tea for at least twenty minutes at a time is very soothing. Sit in a few inches of it in the bath or soak your nether regions in a (clean) washing up bowl.
- Sit in just-warm water, especially if the pain or itching flare up badly in the middle of the night, which they often do.
- Aromatherapists suggest adding ten drops of essential oil of rosemary and ten of tea tree to a just-warm bath to help ease the stinging and itching. Sit in it for 20 minutes.
- Be your own homeopath and try four times daily for up to two weeks:

  Calcarea 6c if itchiness is worse immediately before/after your menstrual period.

Rhus tox 6c if your vulva is very red; but heat makes the itching feel better.

Sulphyr 6 if your vulva is very itchy and your crotch sweaty and smelly. Made worse by heat/washing.

However, for best results see a homeopath for a customised medication.

EAT YOURSELF BETTER

Researchers at the Long Island Jewish Medical Center found in 1992 that if women eat 8oz of live, acidophilus-containing yoghurt a day there is an eighty-five per cent drop in their level of thrush infections. Put the stuff on salads as a dressing with garlic and black pepper, on muesli, on wholewheat pasta as a sauce base, in baked potatoes, or chop fruit into it and have a hip yog-fruit salad.

THRUSH AND SEX

If women eat 8oz of live, acidophilus-containing yoghurt a day there is an eighty-five per cent drop in their level of thrush infections

Sexy, it isn't. Thrush can make intercourse miserably uncomfortable, if not completely out of the question, as any of the eight out of ten women who develop it at some time in their lives, could tell you. Sexual intercourse when you have thrush redoubles the pain and itching during, and especially afterwards. Suddenly cunnilingus, too, no longer seems an attractive option.

Basically, if you've got thrush, don't have any sort of sex with a partner until you are clear. Get your partner treated too. If he's male, he'll probably be symptom free but he can still keep passing it back to you.

When you are better, if you know you are thrush-prone, always use a little lubricating gel like KY when you have intercourse to avoid abrasion of the delicate vaginal skin membranes. Wear cute cotton pants not crotch-murdering nylon ones. Consider wearing really loose cotton knickers (even men's pants) in the last week before your period if you know that's when you are most thrush-prone; or on long, hot, sticky journeys when you are sitting for many hours. Try to avoid combining getting blind drunk, with super-vigorous sex. Though the two can go gloriously together like cigarettes and booze, both alcohol and rough abrasion of the genitals are top thrush-risk factors.

OPERATION ECO-SYSTEM

Help soothe the sting and itch of thrush by smoothing cooled (refrigerated), plain, live yoghurt on the affected area four times a day – it cools, calms and also contains the bacteria lactobacillus. This tiny organism helps defeat thrush by:

- producing lactic acid which acts like a natural, mild antibiotic and competes with other organisms including candida, for glucose;
- helping rebalance the vagina's mini eco-system by preventing the overgrowth of candida.

If you've got thrush, don't have any sort of sex with a partner until you are clear. Get your partner treated too

Many women douche with the yoghurt, for a couple of weeks if necessary. Others use tampons presoaked in the natural yoghurt with a sprinkling of pure acidophilus powder as a natural internal treatment. Don't do this if you are very sore though, as even putting the tampon in place may abrade the swollen skin and be uncomfortable.

HOW TO NEVER GET THRUSH AGAIN

- Wear cotton underwear.
- Avoid wearing tight jeans, Lycra leggings and labia-hugging nylon pants for more than a couple of hours at a time. French knickers (camiknickers) – you may find you need to wear them pulled an inch or two further down your hips, as the seam where the two parts join can cut into your labia, pushing its protective wings of flesh apart, and abrading the delicate tissue inside.
- Use sanitary towels and change them frequently instead of using tampons, which can leach moisture from the vaginal wall leaving it more vulnerable to infection.
- During a period, wash your vulva in cool water each time you change your sanitary towel, because thrush fungi thrive on the nutritionally rich mix of vaginal blood and sweat.
- Use a slick of petroleum gel to protect your vulval skin during,

and for a couple of days after, your period.

- Cut back on anything with refined sugars, refined carbohydrates, alcohol – and very sweet fruit like grapes. Yeast organisms love sugar.
- If you have to take a course of antibiotics, ask for a thrush pessary e.g. Canesten or a Diflucan tablet (a one-off oral treatment), or apply natural yoghurt/lactobacillus powder daily as a thrush-preventing measure. You can take lactobacillus powder internally too – three capsules or a quarter of a teaspoon three times daily should do the trick.
- Avoid perfumed soap and bubble baths and use non biological washing powders for your knickers.

A CLOVE A DAY KEEPS THRUSH AWAY

Thrush hates garlic, as many clinical trials show. If you like the taste of garlic, chew a raw clove of it every day. If you don't, or fear your breath may pong, take 900mg daily of the odour-controlled, coated capsules or tablets which have a standardised allicin (garlic's active ingredient) content, such as the Kwai brand.

TOOTHACHE AND TEETHING

Toothache can vary from the niggling tweak you get when a piece of marshmallow gets caught on a sensitive area, to the sudden onset of blinding, all-encompassing pain from a really feisty abscess on a nerve root. Most lie somewhere in between the two and are the result of:

- tooth decay
- gingivitis
- sensitive teeth
- receding gums which expose a small part of the root (dentists call this 'sensitivity at the gum line', and it makes you jump if cool air or substances touch it)
- neuralgia

- sinusitis, because the pain can be referred
- inflammation of the living tooth pulp, or nerve root.

KILL THE PAIN – YES, YOU CAN

Toothache is usually a sign that you need to visit the dentist as soon as possible. Sadly there is no way around that. Toothache does not go away on its own, or not for long anyway. Ignore intermittent pain, or dowse it down with self-help measures and forget it and it will, as surely as day follows night, make a comeback soon. It will usually do this, Sod's Law being what it is, at a far less convenient time (usually a Sunday, a Bank Holiday or a weekend away).

Toothache does not go away on its own

However, until you get an appointment, there are several temporary, effective comfort measures.

DAB-IT-ON: INSTANT PAIN-STOPPERS: TRY –

- Using a cotton bud to dab tincture of echinacea, or myrrh, or oil of cloves directly on to the area. They are all anaesthetic and anti-infective agents.
- Applying a drop or two of Rescue Remedy, from the Bach Flower range, on to the spot.
- Softening a whole clove – yes, those spiky things you stick in baked hams – and place it in your mouth over the affected area.
- Apply some aloe vera gel on to the area that hurts. According to Seattle dentist Rick Chavez this can temporarily relieve certain types of toothache pain in fifteen minutes flat. This is short-term emergency treatment only – the problem returns after the aloe vera is washed off by saliva.
- Homeopathy can be an effective, rapid emergency treatment for acute conditions as well as a long-term treatment and has been known to stop toothache in its tracks. As a general catch-all treatment, using arnica and hypercium together seems to work well for soothing the aftermath of an extraction, according to Professor Henri Albertini, the assistant dean of the Faculty of Odontology in Marseilles.

These remedies can be tried every 5 minutes (see how you feel after each) for up to 10 doses if you cannot get to see a dentist immediately:

Staphisagria 6 if the toothache's really bad, made worse by cold air, food, and even the lightest pressure, especially if the bad tooth is blackened or your cheek swollen and red.

Belladonna 30 if the pain's best described as throbbing, your mouth's dry and you are developing a gumboil too.

Apis 30 if the pain burns and stings and your gums feel tight and swollen.

Arnica 30 if you are in pain after a filling or having a tooth out. Take as soon as you get home, three times a day for day one, then once a day if needed for the next few days.

- Make a herbal tea from one of the following – hops, valerian, wild lettuce or skullcap – to help ease the pain. You may need to drink the tea throughout the day so make a reasonable quantity – use 1oz of the dried herb in a pint of boiling water, let it steep for three to four minutes, drain, and drink a teacupful at a time.

Acupuncture can be effective enough for dentists to use as their only form of anaesthesia when extracting teeth

PRESS HERE

Acupuncture can be effective enough for dentists to use as their only form of anaesthesia when extracting teeth. You can sometimes use acupressure (acupuncture minus needles) to help deal with toothache until you can see the dentist. Try the general painkilling point L Hegu 4. It is in the web of fleshy skin between your index finger and thumb. Feel around there for the most sensitive point. Rotate the ball of your thumb on that spot firmly for about four minutes, take a twenty-minute break and repeat as necessary.

For emergency DIY acupressure press the pressure points on both sides of the mouth just where the lips meet. Press the pressure points on either side of the nose at their widest point (junction between nose and cheeks). Do so for three minutes each, say half an hour apart (see diagram p. 137).

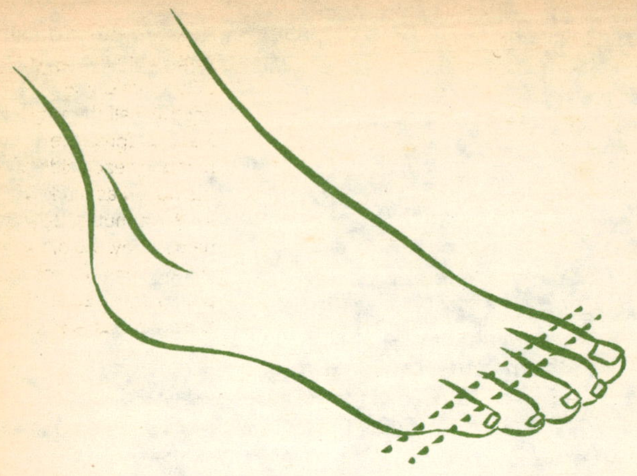

To help soothe toothache and teething pain using reflexology. Press thumb gently along the area marked for 2-3 minutes, every 20 minutes. Do this on both feet.

TOOTHACHE TIP

If you are taking the ordinary ibuprofen as a painkiller, wash it down with a cup of coffee or strong tea. Oxford researchers found that when they tried giving caffeine plus the medicine to a group of people who'd just had their impacted back teeth removed, the drug worked better and faster.

TEETHING

Teething tends to plague babies, toddlers – and their parents – on and off between about four months and three years of age. Teething pain is the discomfort and inflammation produced when a baby's first teeth begin to push their way up through the surface of their gums.

Symptoms can include pain and aching either locally or around the entire jaw area, sometimes producing earache as well, a temperature and mild diarrhoea – though some children do not seem too bothered and the only sign of teething is some spectacular dribbling. However, if anything is going to be uncomfortable for them, it is usually their front incisors which tend to come through first, and

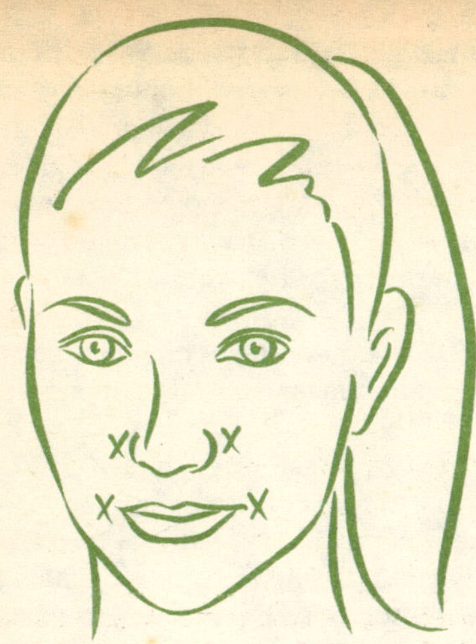

To ease toothache, try gently stimulating what traditional Chinese doctors call the Ying Xiang acupressure points by each side of the nostril as marked for 2-3 minutes, 2-3 times a day. Also, try stimulating the Dicong points at the edge of the mouth as marked.

parents anecdotally report that these teeth seem to be the sorest.

Mothers and fathers usually know instinctively if their child is uncomfortable or unhappy, but apart from crying, restlessness and grizzling, babies make it plain they are teething by several other signs, including fist-chewing, dribbling, a raised temperature, a red patch on one or both cheeks, rattiness and disturbed sleep (yours, and theirs).

Unfortunately you can't make the teeth come through faster, but you can do an enormous amount to help soothe any discomfort they are causing. The three things which seem to help any discomfort while they do so are chewing, distraction, and natural pain-soothing medicines and massages.

THINGS TO CHEW ON

- Clean, chilled plastic teething rings. Put them in the freezer for ten minutes beforehand – but no longer or they can cause ice burns on top of everything else. Buy three or four (they are very cheap) and keep a constant supply handy.
- You can do the same with apple or carrot slices, if your child is old enough.
- Slow-baked thick slices of bread make great (cheap, sugar-free) rusks for a child to gnaw on.

WHAT SOOTHES TEETHING DISCOMFORT

- Aroma-soother. A soothing aromatherapy rub on the outside of the affected cheek. Use two drops of Roman chamomile (it is said to have anti-inflammatory properties) essential oil in a palmful of sweet almond oil. Alternatively add a single drop to an egg cup full of cold water, dip in a cotton wool bud and apply gently to the baby's gums. Keep this in the fridge for up to 24 hours to use whenever you need it.
- Chamomile tea: use one teaspoon of the herb in half a pint of boiling water, let it steep for four minutes, strain and use. If they are happy to drink it from a bottle or feeding cup, so much the better. If not, make a cool compress out of the tea and lay it against their sore cheek.
- Homeopathy can be very effective for teething. Try Nelsons homeopathic teething granules (a general, catch-all remedy you can buy in the health food shop or some chemists) as a starter, but it will be more effective if you can match the homeopathic medication more closely to the type of teething discomfort your baby is having. Try:

  Mercurius 6 if they have sore gums, some diarrhoea and are dribbling freely.

  Aconite 30 if they are in obvious pain and running a temperature.

  Chamomilla 30 if they just want to be carried around by you all the time, cry louder when put down, are irritable and have one red cheek.

  Try the remedies every 30 minutes (more often if your child is in acute discomfort) for up to 10 doses, suggests homeopathic GP Dr Andrew Lockie.

  One piece of German research carried out on forty-two toddlers in 1994 (average age nearly sixteen months) found that homeopathic treatment worked well for eighty-three per cent of them.

SUCKLING SWEETNESS SOOTHES PAIN

When babies suckle on a bottle or breast, they trigger the release of their own natural painkilling chemicals, according to new research at the University of Maryland Dental School in Baltimore, 1997. Apparently the sweetness of breast milk boosts the effect – so if your baby is bottle fed, sweeten it slightly or let them have slightly sweet-tasting diluted juice when they need a natural teething pain cure.

DISTRACTION

Carry your baby around in a sling for as long as possible if this is what seems to comfort them – the motion of your walking and their snuggled closeness to you, and their changing view of the world as you move around will all help. If they are screaming too hard for this, take them out in their pram or buggy. Singing to them, playing music to them and quietly reading to them and showing them a picture book all act as effective, gentle distractions – babies like looking at books from a very early age and certainly by four to six months. They like the sound of your voice even better.

VARICOSE VEINS

Varicose veins don't look too pretty, and they can be painful. Usually varicose veins develop in the legs and become distended, sometimes lengthened, even twisted and 'knotted', but can also affect the rectum, where they are better known as haemorrhoids, or piles. They may also appear around the vulva during pregnancy too, though fortunately this type tends to disappear soon after you have had your baby.

Varicose veins develop when blood flow trying to return to the heart is obstructed in some way, usually when something is squashing nearby blood vessels. In pregnancy that something is the increasing weight of your growing baby, in non-pregnancy the cause is often traced to the rectum and to constipation, or to a general weakness in the valves inside the veins whose job it is to prevent blood flowing backwards.

Varicose veins tend to run in families where there is an inherited weakness in the blood vessel walls or valves

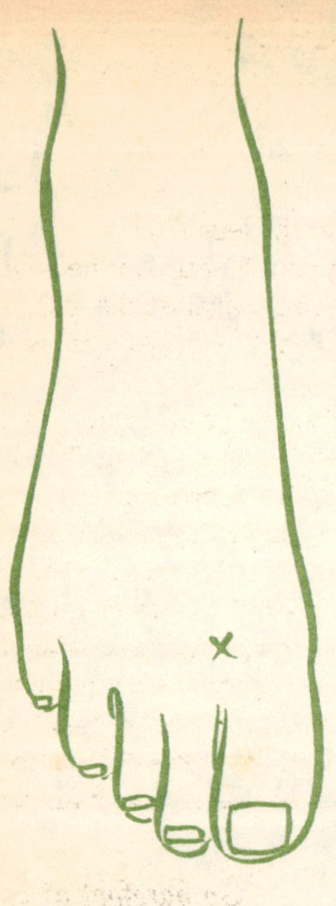

For helping to relieve the ache of varicose veins, and also help prevent them in the first place. This is the Liver 3 acupressure point. You can find it on the top of the foot, just down from the web between the first and second toes. Gently press here with your thumb in the hollow between the bones/tendons for between 30 seconds and 2 minutes. This helps increase circulation in the toes, helps prevent varicose veins, and relieves aching.

Varicose veins may be thoroughly uncomfortable, they may be purely cosmetic (unsightly 'grape-vine' veins, or flare veins) but if the problem has developed in a vein that is buried deep in the body tissue, this can cause a throbbing and aching in the calves, leg swelling, purpling and discolouring of the skin in the area, dry, flaky irritable skin (varicose eczema) and ulcers. Varicose veins tend to run in families where there is an inherited weakness in the blood vessel walls or valves. If you are overweight, constipated, take little exercise or have to stand up a lot, these factors make the veins worse.

Longer term, the anti-varicose veins plan includes plenty of fibre in your diet, drinking at least three pints of plain water daily to tackle constipation, and exercise to gee up circulation. It does not have to be much – a brisk walk for fifteen minutes a day is fine, says specialist venous surgeon Dr Robert May of the University of Innsbruck in Austria. Nutritionists suggest upping your intake of vitamins E and C, and of bioflavonoids too.

TAKING THE THROB OUT OF VARICOSE VEINS

- Hot and cold water splashed over the legs.
- When you can, lie down and put your feet up on the sofa arm or cushion, or even lie with your bottom against the wall and your legs leaning up against it at as near ninety degrees as you can manage.
- Wear support tights – Boots has some good quality ones which simply look like ordinary opaque fashion tights, in slimming dark colours (black, navy, bottle green, iron grey etc.)
- Add five drops of essential oil of cypress to your bath. Don't have the water too hot as this will make the veins throb even more.
- Massage the vein area with a palmful of carrier oil and three drops of cypress and three drops of lavender essential oil, using strokes flowing up towards the heart only, three times a week.
- Bathe the veins in witch hazel as this can be cooling and soothing.
- Bathe the veins in cold (from the fridge) comfrey tea. Use l oz of the herb to one pint of boiling water, or a teaspoonful per cup of boiling water. Stir well and let it steep for ten minutes. Strain, cool and use.
- For the relief of really bad aching wipe with a cotton cloth containing crushed ice for a few seconds.
- Try homeopathy, for example:

  H*amamelis* 30*c* if the vein area feels sore and bruised, and you also, on top of everything else, have piles.

  F*errum* 30*c* if your legs are aching and weak but walking helps the feeling wear off slowly, and if they are usually quite pale but go red easily.

  Take these remedies every twelve hours for up to a week. If there is no improvement after three weeks or matters take a turn for the worse, see your GP.

> *Go barefoot at home or on the beach as much as possible. Work at Innsbruck University suggests this exercises the foot muscles and helps the venous flow in the legs*

Do:

Go barefoot at home or on the beach as much as possible. Work at Innsbruck University suggests this exercises the foot muscles and helps the venous flow in the legs.

Don't:

Read on the loo, or sit there for hours straining. Research at Oxford's John Radcliffe Hospital in 1989 backs up the old wives tale about reading on the loo. Men especially should be discouraged from disappearing in there with the newspaper in the mornings. Not only is it anti-social, loo-hogging, washing up-avoiding behaviour but research confirms you're also more likely to get piles.

PREGNANCY TIP

If you are pregnant, wear support tights from the fourth month – do not wait for your legs to start aching. Put the tights on *before* you get up out of bed in the morning, keeping them under your pillow or in the bedside drawer. They're not much help if you put them on after you've swung your feet on to the floor as the blood will pool in your feet/ankles/legs under gravity's pull, right away.

GETTING HELP

HELPLINES

Arthritis Care, 18 Stephenson Way, London NW1 2HD. Tel: 0171 916 1505.

The British Dietetic Association, 5th Floor, Elizabeth House, 22 Suffolk Street, Queensway, Birmingham, B1 1LS. Tel: 0121 616 4900. This is the professional body for private nutritionists who have had the 3-year training course that's recognised by the NHS. Fees payable. You can also ask your GP to refer you to an NHS nutritionist, though waiting lists may be long due to NHS cutbacks.

British Association of Autogenic Training and Therapy, Heath Cottage, Pitch Hill, Ewhurst, Nr Cranleigh, Surrey, GU6 7NP.

The Campaign to Legalise Cannabis International Association, 54c Peacock Street, Norwich NR3 lTB.

CHICK (Cannabis Help Information Club), PO Box 2223, Glastonbury, BA6 9YU. Organisation whose activities include, amongst other things, sending (free of charge) small amounts of cannabis to be used for medicinal purposes by people who are chronically ill. At the time of writing was still solvent and functioning.

Cystitis? by Angela Kilmartin. After reading this book if you still need additional advice write (enclosing an sae) to its author, an anti-cystitis campaigning veteran, at 75 Mortimer Road, London N1 5AR.

The Food Intolerance Data Bank. Tel: 01372 376 761. Fax: 01372 386 228. Product information about the foods that may be associated with intolerance or allergy – useful for those suffering certain types of chronic pain as many such conditions (including arthritis, rheumatism, IBS) have links with certain foods. Information is only available to medical practitioners so members of the public are not allowed to call the data bank direct – ask your GP to fax for you.

The Herpes Viruses Association, 41 North Road, London N7 9DP. Helpline: 0171 609 9061.

Homeopaths – to find a medically qualified homeopath i.e. one who is also a medical doctor, contact The British Homeopathic Association, 27a Devonshire Street, London, W1N 1RJ. Tel: 0171 935 2163. For a lay (non-medically qualified but professionally trained) homeopath, contact The Society of Homeopaths, 2 Artizan Road, Northampton, NN1 3HR. Tel: 01604 621 400.

Independent Midwives Association. Tel: 01344 396 409. Professionally trained midwives who now work outside the NHS and are very sympathetic to natural/active childbirth practices, including natural methods of pain relief. For a list of members send an sae to the IMA Register, 94 Auckland Road, Upper Norwood, London SE19.

Institute for Complementary Medicine, PO Box 194, London SE16 7QZ. Tel: 0171 237 5165. Has its own register of good, professional therapists around the UK who practice the different forms of complementary medicine, from AK to Shiatsu.

The Medical Alliance for Cannabis Therapeutics, PO Box CR14, Leeds LS7 4XS. Fax 01532 371 000.

Migraine Action Association, 178a High Road, West Byfleet, Surrey KT14 7ED. Tel: 01932 352 468.

The National Back Pain Association, 16 Elmtree Road, Teddington,

Middlesex TW11 8ST. Tel: 0181 977 5474.

National Childbirth Trust, Alexandra House, Oldham Terrace, London W3 6NH. Tel: 0181 992 8637. Advice, help and support on all aspects of pregnancy, childbirth and breastfeeding.

National Register of Hypnotherapists and Psychotherapists, for information send an sae to 12 Cross Street, Nelson, Lancashire, BB9 7EN tel: 01282 699 378. The register has a list of countrywide members – all are psychotherapists who are also qualified in hypnotherapy.

The National Sports Medicine Institute, Charterhouse Square, London EC1M 6BQ. The Institute has a list of accredited sports injury clinics countrywide.

Painwise UK, 33 Kingsdown Park, Tankerton, Kent CT5 2DT. Tel: 01227 277 993. A self-help organisation for people who live with chronic pain of all types.

RSI (Repetitive Strain Injury) Association, 380–384 Harrow Road, London W9 2HU. Tel: 0171 266 2000

The Shingles Support Society, 41 North Road, London N7. Tel: 0171 609 9061.

The Women's Nutritional Advisory Service, PO Box 268, Lewes, East Sussex, BN7 2QN. Tel: 01273 487 366.

BOOKS WHICH TELL YOU MORE

Acupressure Step by Step by Jackeline Young, Thorsons, 1998, £9.99.

The Family Guide to Homeopathy by Dr Andrew Lockie, Hamish Hamilton, 1998, £15.99. See also the website www.drlockie.com

In Pain? by Dr Chris Wells and Graham Nown, Optima, 1993, £7.99.

Pain Relief in Childbirth by Nikki Bradford and Geoffrey Chamberlain, HarperCollins, 1995, £6.99.

What They Don't Tell You About Being a Mother and Having Babies by Nikki Bradford and Jean Williams, HarperCollins, 1997, £12.99.

SHOPPING GUIDE – WHERE DO I GET IT FROM?

The Active Birth Centre. Tel: 0171 561 9006. Runs active birth courses around the country teaching natural and active childbirth techniques, relaxation/visualisation, yoga for pregnancy and birth, and hires out water pools.

Ainsworths Homeopathic Pharmacy, 36 New Cavendish Street, London W1. Tel: 0171 935 5330. Good advice from trained homeopathic staff over the phone, and prompt mail-order service of homeopathic remedies and tinctures.

Back-friendly chairs, desks, beds, massagers, neck rests – you name it, from: **The Back Shop**. Tel: 0171 935 9120.

Bio-force: Good range of herbal tinctures, such as echinacea and hypericum. Stocked in major health shops.

Culpeper's the Herbalists: several shops around the UK but has a mail-order service for its good-quality range of dried traditional herbs and aromatherapy oils. Tel: 01223 894 054.

Eladon: makers of Elagen supplement, Bangor, North Wales. Tel: 01248 370 054.

Ergonomic Keyboards: PCD Maltron Ltd, 15 Orchard Lane, East Molesey, Surrey. Tel: 0181 398 3265.

Gerrard House (aromatherapy oils) English Grains Healthcare, William Nadin

Way, Swadlincote DE11 0BB. Consumer helpline: 01283 228 344.

Hands-free computing equipment: (voice-response etc) Hands Free Computing Ltd, 1a Windsor Road, Wraybury, Staines, Middx. Tel: 01784 483 824.

Hands-free headsets: Plantronics Headsets, Plantronics Ltd, Interface Business Park, Bincknoll Lane, Wootton Bassett, Wiltshire. Tel: 01793 842 200.

The Health and Diet Company (FSC Vitamins), Unit E1, Europa Park, Stoneclough Road, Radcliffe, Manchester M26 1GG. Tel: 01204 707 420. A very wide range of good quality vitamin, mineral, and nutritional, and herbal supplements and herbal teas (the Herbcraft range is available in tincture, spray and tablet form). Rapid mail-order service available, also information on your nearest local supplier of specific products. Advice over the phone concerning their specific supplements and products. Can also provide information on medical trials carried out on the vitamins, herbal tinctures, minerals and supplements they supply, where available.

Helios Homeopathics (homeopathic pharmacy), 89-95 Camden Road, Tunbridge Wells, Kent TN1 2QR. Tel: 01892 537 254. Has very good, rapid mail order service and homeopaths can give advice about the remedies over the phone – they send you the remedy express and you pay when you receive it.

Milk for the lactose-intolerant: Lactolite (Lactolite Info Bureau), MD Foods Plc, Craven House, Kirkstall Road, Leeds LS3 1JE.

Nature's Best: PO Box 1, Tunbridge Wells, Kent TW2 3EQ. Tel: 01892 552 118. Good range of vitamin, mineral and nutritional supplements. Available mail order, or from health food shops.

Neal's Yard Remedies: mail-order line: 0161 831 7875. Extensive and good-quality range of traditional loose and dried medicinal herbs and powders; aromatherapy oils and health books on the therapies concerned. Reliable advice given over the phone and in their shops about the products they have.

Solgar Vitamins, Aldbury, Tring, Hertfordhire HP23 5PT. Tel: 01442 890355. The company's Gold Label range includes more than 250 high-quality vitamins, minerals, herbs, amino acids and food supplements and they are sold in health shops UK wide (and in 38 other countries as well). Most of the nutrients and herbs they offer have often been used in clinical trials worldwide. There is no mail-order service but Solgar can tell you which health shops in your area stock the products you are looking for, and can also give advice about the supplements' use over the phone. Can also provide, on special request, clinical trial information to confirm that certain supplements do indeed work.

Splashdown, 1 Wellington Terrace, Harrow on the Hill, Midddlesex. Tel: 0181 422 9308. Rents and delivers birthing pools for use at home or in hospital from around £160. Tip: If you are going to have your baby in hospital and you'd like to use a water pool, check first with the head of Midwifery Services, to see whether they already have one on site, or whether there is space for you to bring your own in and if that's OK with the midwifery staff.

TENS machines: available on a free three week trial so that you can see if they work well enough before buying your own, from Eastwood and Eastwood Ltd, 113 East Barnet Road, Barnet, Herts EM4 8RE. Tel. 0181 441 9641.

Vitamin amounts ... what's in your bottle of pills? The way in which amounts of vitamin A, beta-carotene, vitamins D, E and C are expressed on supplements' labels is changing, eg vitamin E used to be 'iu', now 'mg'. Check with retailer, manufacturer or nutritionist if confused.

RESEARCH REFERENCES ... WHO SAYS THESE THINGS WORK ANYWAY?

WHAT IS PAIN?

Laughter: 'The Effects of Laughter and Relaxation on Discomfort Thresholds' by R. and D. Cogan and W. Walz, in the *Journal of Behavioural Medicine* 1987 (2); 'Laughter decreases cortisol, epinephrine, and 3,4 – dihydroyphenenyl acetic acid' by L.S. Berk, L.A. Tan et al in *Abstract of Behavioural Medicine* 1988.

WHICH COMPLEMENTARY THERAPY FOR SELF HELP

Reflexology: Postal workers: in *Zoneterapeuter* Nov 1993, by S. Masden, J. Andersen et al. Childbirth: unpublished study by Dr Gowri Motha and Dr Jane McGrath. *Pain Relief in Childbirth* by N. Bradford and G. Chamberlain, 1995. Acupressure: back pain: *The Journal of Traditional Chinese Medicine*, 1986, vol 6 (3) by W. Jiaying, L. Guangzhoa et al. Homeopathy: Migraines: double blind trial: *The Berlin Journal on Research in Homeopathy*, March 1991, vol 1, no 2, by B. Brigo, G. Serpelloni et al. See Breast pain and Toothache sections, trials using homeopathy. Colour therapy: *Mind Bulletin* vol 15, no 4, Jan 1990, by J. Anderson. Arthritis: *International Journal of Biosocial Research* vol 3, no 2, 1982, by S.F. McDonald. Relaxation and Visualisation: for IBS: *Journal of Advanced Nursing*, 1986, vol 11, no 65, by B. Milne, G. Joachim et al. For headaches; *International Journal of Clinical Hypnosis*, Jan 1991, vol 39 (1) by R. Van Dyke and F.G. Zitman. Painful aspects of Raynaud's Disease: *Journal of Applied Behaviour Analysis*, 1980 vol 13 (1), F.J. Keefe et al.

ARTHRITIS AND RHEUMATISM

Avoiding solanine in foods: 'A Relationship of Arthritis to Solanaceae (nightshades)', by N.F. Childrers, in the *Journal of Interact. Acad. Pre. Med*, Nov 1982. Allergy links: with RA: 'Placebo Controlled, Double Blind Study of Dietary Manipulation Therapy in Rheumatoid Arthritis', by L.G. Darlington, N.W. Ramsey et al, *Lancet*, 1986, I; 'The Effect of Dietary Restrictions on Disease Activity in Rheumatoid Arthritis', by D. Beri et al, *Annals of Rheumatic Diseases*, 1988, vol 47; 'Possible Role of Food Sensitivity in Arthritis', by R.S. Panush, Annals of Allergy, 1988, 61 (part 2); 'Food Allergy as an Etiological Factor in Anthropathies: a survey' by M.R. Taylor, in the *Journal of Interact. Acad. Prev. Med.* 1983, vol 8; 'Diets for Rheumatoid Arthritis', by L.G. Darlington and N.W. Ramsey, *Lancet*, 1991m 338. The Warmbrand Diet: *How Thousands of my Arthritis Patients Regained their Health*, M. Warmbrand, Acro Publishing, 1974. Vit C: 'Do Anti-oxidant Micronutrients Protect against the Development and Progression of Knee Arthritis?' by McAlidon et al, in *Arthritis and Rheumatism*, 1996, 39 (4). Vitamin E: 'Tocopheraol in Osteoarthritis: a controlled pilot study', by I Machtey et al, in the *Journal of the American Geriatric Society*, 1978 (25). Fish oils for OA: 'Inflammation in osteoarthritis' by R. Altman and R. Gray, *Clin. Rheum. Dis.*, 1985 (11). Boron: 'Boron and Arthritis: the results of a double blind pilot study' by R.L. Travers et al, *J. Nutr. Med.*, 1990, I. 'The role of boron in human nutrition', by R.E. Newnham, *J of Appl.*

Nutrition, 1994, 46. Glucosamine sulfate for RA: 'Therapeutic Activity of Oral Glucosamine Sulphate in the Management of Osteoarthritis of the knee in out-patients' by A.L. Vaz, in *Curr. Med. Res. Opin.*, 1982, 8 (3); 'Double Blind Clinical Evaluation of Oral Glucosamine Sulphate in the Basic Treatment of Osteoarthrosis', by J.M. Pujalte et al; 'Therapeutic Activity of Oral Glucosamine Sulphate in Osteoarthritis: a placebo-controlled, double-blind investigation', by A. Drovanti et al, *Clin. Ther.* 1980 (4). GLA (Evening primrose oil, starflower oil, borage) helping reduce inflammation of arthritis: *The Scandinavian Journal of Rheumatology*, 1983, vol 12, pp 85-8; *The British Journal of Rheumatology*, 1991, vol 30, 370-2. 'Treatment of Rheumatoid Arthritis with GLA' by L.J. Leventhal et al, *The Annals of Internal Medicine*, 1993, vol 119. 'Evening Primrose Oil in Patients with Rheumatoid Arthritis' by M. Brzenski et al, *British Journal of Rheumatology*, 1991, vol 30. Acupuncture: 'Efficacy of Traditional Chinese Acupuncture in the Treatment of Symptomatic Knee Osteoarthritis: a pilot study', by A.K. McIndoe and K. Young, in *Osteoarthritis and Cartilage*, 1995, vol 3; 'Acupuncture for the Treatment of Pain in Osteoarthritic Knees' by W. Takeda and J. Wessel, *Arthritis Care and Research*. White Willow: 'Herbal Medicine' by R.F. Weiss, Gothenberg, Sweden, *Ab Arcanum*, 1988, vol 31; *The British Herbal Compendium*, ed by P.R. Bradley, vol 1, published by the British Herbal Medicine Association, 1992. Burdock root: *The Herbal Handbook: A User's Guide to Medical Herbalism* by D. Hoffman, Healing Arts Press, 1988 pp 23-4. Special eating plans (low fat/vegetarian, gluten free): 'Dietary Fat Aggravates Rheumatoid Arthritis', by C.P. Lucas et al, *Clin. Res*, 1981, 29; 'Fasting and Vegan Diet in Rheumatoid Arthritis', by L Skolsdtram, *Scandinavian Journal of Rheumatology*, 1987, vol 15; 'Effects of Uncooked Vegan Food – "living food" – on Rheumatoid Arthritis, a three month controlled and randomised study', by M. Nenonen et al, *The American Journal of Clinical Nutrition*, 1992, vol 56; 'Controlled Trial of Fasting and One Year Vegetarian Diet in Rheumatoid Arthritis', by Kjeldsen-Kragh, *Lancet*, 1991, 338. Gold rings: '*Annals of Rheumatic Diseases*' 1997. Copper: 'An Investigation into the Therapeutic Value of the "copper bracelet". Dermal Assimilation of Copper in Arthritic/rheumatric Conditions', by W.R. Walker et al, *Agents Actions*, 1976, vol 6; 'Copper, Iron, Free Radicals and Arthritis' by D.R. Blake et al, in the *British Journal of Rheumatology*, 1985; 'Copper Boosts the Activity of Anti-inflammatory Drugs', by J.R.J. Sorenson, in *Progress Med. Chem.* 1978, vol 15. Yucca plants: 'Yucca Plant Saponin in the Management of Arthritis', by R. Bingham et al, the *Journal of Applied Nutrition*, 1975, vol 27; '*A Field Guide to Medicinal Plants: Eastern and Central North America*', by S. Fosters and J.A. Duke, Houghton Mifflin Co, Boston, 1990. Homeopathy: 'Homeopathic Therapy in Rheumatoid Arthritis: Evaluation by Double Blind Clinical Trial', by R.G. and S.L.M. Gibson et al, the *British Journal of Clinical Pharmacology*, 1980, vol 9. Selenium for RA: 'Low Selenium Levels in Severe Rheumatoid Arthritis', by Tarp, Overvad et al, *Scandinavian Journal of Rheumatology*, 1985, vol 14. Vit E: 'Treatment of Rheumatoid Arthritis with Selenium and Vit E', by Munthe and Aseth, *Scandinavian Journal of Rheumatology*, 1984, vol 53. Zinc: 'Treatment of Rheumatoid Arthritis with Oral Zinc Sulphate', by P.A. Simkin, in *Agents and Actions* (supplement) 1981, vol 8. Vit C: 'New Concepts in Biology and Biochemistry of Ascorbic Acid', by M. Levine, *The New England Journal of Medicine* 1986, vol 314. Feverfew: 'Extracts of Feverfew Inhibit Granule Secretion in Blood Platelets and Plymorphonuclear Leucocytes', by S. Heptinstasll et al, *Lancet*, 1985. Devils Claw as an anti-inflammatory: *Handbook of Medicinal Herbs*, by J.A. Duke, Boca Raton Press, 1985; *Encyclopedia of Common Natural Ingredients Used in Food, Drugs and Cosmetics* by A.Y. Leung, John Wiley and Sons, New York, 1980. Reflexology: paper presented by Guang-Ming, at the Shenzhen City, China, Reflexology Symposium, July 1993. Paper by the Australian Association of Reflexologists, Feb 1994, in the Australian ICR (Int. Comms. Refl) Newsletter. Cannabis: oncologists survey in US: 'Marijuana as Anti-emetic Medicine' by R.E. Doblin and M.A. Kleinman, the Kennedy School of Govt, *Cambridge Journal of Clin Oncol.*, Nov 1991; 'Effects of IV THC* on Experimental and Surgical Pain', by D. Raft and J. Gregg, Clib, *Pharm and Therapeutics*, 21 Jan 1977; 'Marijuana Changes in Pain Tolerance', by S.L. Milstein and K. MacCannell, *International Pharmacopsychiatry*, 1975, 10 (3); 'Effects of Moderate and High Doses of Marijuana on Thermal Pain', by W.C. Clark and M.N. Janal, *Journal of Clinical Pharmacology*, 1981 Aug/Sept. Cannabis and MS: 'The Perceived Effects of Smoked Cannabis on Patients with MS', by P. Consroe and R. Musty et al, *European Neurology*, 1997, vol 33 (1); 'The Analgesic Effect of Delta-9 THC', by R.J. Noyes, S. Brunk et al, in the *Journal of Clinical Pharmacology*, 1995, No 15, pp 139-43. (* THC is the active ingredient in cannabis)

BACK PAIN

Acupuncture: an overview look at several papers on back pain and acupuncture: 'Randomised Controlled Trials of Acupuncture for Back Pain – a Meta Analysis' by A.R. White and E. Ernst, 1977 – in preparation at time of writing, details from the British Medical Acupuncture Society. White Willow: 'Herbal Medicine' by R.F. Weiss, Gothenberg, Sweden, *Ab Arcanum* 1988, vol 31; *The British Herbal Compendium*, ed by P.R. Bradley, vol 1, published by the British Medical Herbalism Association, 1992. Reflexology: paper by Kovacs, Abraira, Copez-Abente and Poeg, in *Medicina Clinica* 1993, vol 101.

BREAST PAIN

Caffeine: 'The effects of Caffeine Free Diet on Benign Breast Disease: A Randomised Trial', *Surgery*, vol 91, by V.L. Ernster et al, no. 3 1982; 'Caffeine, Cyclic Mastalgia and Breast Disease', *Surgery*, vol 86 1979, by J.P. Minton et al. Evening Primrose Oil (EPO): 'Clinical Experience of Drug Treatments for Mastalgia', *Lancet* vol 2, 1985, J.K. Pye et al; 'The Effects of Essential Fatty Acids on Cyclical Mastalgia' by R.E. Mansel, J.K. Pye et al, *Omega Essential Fatty Acids*, published by Alan R. Liss, NY, 1990. Vitamins E and A: 'The Role of Vitamin E in Fibrocystic Breast Disease', in *Obstetrics and Gynaecology* vol 65 1982 by R.S. London et al; 'The Use of Vitamin E for Chronic Cystic Mastitis', The *New England Journal of Medicine*, vol 272, 1965, by A.A. Abrahams. Iodine: 'Mammary Gland Dysplasia in Iodine Deficiency', by B.A. Eskin et al, *Journal of the American Medical Association*, vol 200, 1967. Low-fat diet: 'Effect of a Low-fat Diet on Hormone Levels of Women with Cystic Breast Disease' by D.P. Rose, A.P. Boyar and C. Cohen, JNCI, 1987, vol 78; 'Effect of Low-fat, High-carbohydrate Diet on Symptoms of Clinical Mastopathy', by N.F. Boyd and V. McGuire, *Lancet* 1988, ii. Agnus-Castus (Vittex): 'Agnus Castus Extacts Inhibit Prolactin Secretion of Rat Pituitary Cells', by G. Skliutz and P. Speiser et al, in *Horm Metab Res*, 1993, Vol 25. Homeopathy: 'Essai Therapeutique en Homeopathie Traitment des Tensions Mammaires et Mastodynies du Syndrome Premenstruel', C. Lepaisant, *Rev. Fr Gynecol Obstet*, 1995, 90; 2, 94-7. 'Expansion Scientifique Francaise, 1995'.

BUNIONS

For anti-inflammatory effects of GLA, fish oils, bosweilla, white willow, cayenne etc see Arthritis section.

CHILDBIRTH

Acupuncture: *The Midwives Chronicle* 1988; *Anaesthesia and Analgesia* 1975, *The American Journal of Chinese Medicine*, 1977; The Report on Acupuncture and Childbirth at the 1978 International Conference on Acupuncture in Sri Lanka. Pain: *Akush Ginekol Mosk* (1984) and *Anesteziol Reanimatol*: papers by Koraeva, Ustinova and Poliuanova, 1980; *The Midwives Chronicle* 1988; *Anaesthesia and Analgesia* 1975; *The American Journal of Chinese Medicine*, 1977; *The Report on Childbirth at the* 1978 *International Conference on Acupuncture in* Sri *Lanka*. Reflexology: paper by Sakala in *Social Science Medicine* 1988, vol 22.

CRAMP

Homeopathy: 'A Study in the Effectiveness of Ultra-low Doses of Copper in the Treatment of Hemodialysis-related Muscle Cramps' by E. Hariveau, P. Nolen et al, *Ultra Low Doses* ed by C. Doutremepuich, published by Talyor-Franic of London, 1991.

CYSTITIS

Cranberry juice:' Reduction of Bacteria and Pyuria after Ingestion of Cranberry Juice' by J. Avron, M. Monane, J.H. Gurwitz et al, *Journal of the American Medical Association* (JAMA) 1994, 271. 'Inhibition of Adherence by Cranberry Juice' A.E. Sobota, *The Journal of Urology*, 1984, 131. Sugar, fats and alcohol: 'Role of Sugars in Human Neutrophilic Phagocytosis' by Sanchez and Reeser, in *The American Journal of Clinical Nutrition*, 1971, vol 26; 'Alcohol and Immune Defence', R.R. MacGregor, JAMA, 1986, 256 (ll); 'Dietary fat and Natural Killer-cell Activity' by J. Barone et al; *Am J. of Cl Nut*, 1989, 50; Allergies: 'Allergy and Infection', by A.J. Horesh, *Journal of Asthma Res*, 1967, Vol 4. 'Pseudomononucleosis of Allergic Origin: a New Clinical Entity', B.A. Berman in *The Annals of Allergy*, 1964, vol 22; 'The Co-incidence of Allergic Disease, Unexplained Fatigue and Lymphadenopathy' by T.G. Randolph and R.A. Hettig in the *American Journal of Medical Science*, 1945, vol 209. 'Ascorbic Acid and Urinary PH' by D.R. Axelrod, JAMA, 1985 254 (10). Goldenseal: 'Influence of Berberine Sulphate on Synthesis and Expression of Pap Fimbrial Adhesin in Uropathogenic E. Coli' by D.X. Sun and S.N. Abraham, *Antim. Agents Chemother* 1988, vol 32. Uva Ursi: 'Proposal for European Monographs' by the *European Scientific Co-operative for Phytotherapy*, Vol 3, ESCOP Secretariat, Bevrijdingslaan, The Netherlands, 1992; 'Prophylactic Effects of UVA-E in Women with Recurrent Cystitis' by B. Larsson, A. Johasson et al. Lactobascillus: *Clinical Therapy*, 1992, 14: 11-16. Homeopathy: 'A Clinical Trial of Sataphyysagria in Postcoital Cystitis', by P.A. Ustianowski MRCS, in the *British Journal of Homeopathy*, 1974, 63 (4).

EARACHE

Homeopathy: 'The Homeopathic Treatment of Otitis Media in Children – comparisons with conventional therapy' by K.H. Friese, S. Kruse et al, The *International Journal of Clinical Pharmacology and Therapeutics*, Vol 35, No 7, 1997. 'Zur Behandlung der otitis Media mit Pulsatilla' by V. Paul Mossinger, in *der Kinderartz*, 1985, 16 Jg, Nr. 4.

EYESTRAIN

Acupressure: *Acupuncture Textbook and Atlas* by Gabriel Stux and Bruce Pomeranz published by Springer-Verlang (Berline, Heidelberg, New York, Tokyo) 1986. Eyebright: *Herbs for Common Ailments* by Anne McIntyre, NIMH, published by Gaia 1992; *The Hamlyn Encylopaedia of Complementary Medicine*, ed by Nikki Bradford, 1996, Hamlyn. Homeopathy: *The Family Guide to Homeopathy – the safe form of medicine for the future* by Dr Andrew Lockie, Hamish Hamilton, 1990. *A Modern Herbal* by Mrs A. Grieve (Jonathan Cape 1931, Penguin Handbooks 1984).

FIRST AID: STINGS, BITES, BRUISES, STRAINS, BURNS AND SCALDS

Lavender oil: *The Extra Pharmacopoeia*, by Martindale 1972, pub by The Pharmaceutical Press, 26th ed. Bromelain: 'Control of Swelling in Boxing Injuries' by J. Blonstein, in *Practitioner*, 1960, 203. Arnica: Vit C: 'An effect of Ascorbic Acid on Delayed Muscle Soreness', by M. Kaminski and B. Boal, *Pain* 1992, vol 50. Apis, Echinacea, Ledum and Urtica – homeopathic preparations: 'The Efficacy of Prrrikweg (sic) Gel in the Treatment of Insect Bites: a double blind, placebo controlled clinical trial' by N. Hill et al, London School of Tropical Medicine, *Pharmacy World and Science*, vol 18, No 4, pp 35 +, 1996; also the *European Journal of Clinical Pharmacology*, 1995, 49, 103-8: 'A Placebo Controlled Clinical Trial Investigating the Efficacy of a Homeopathic After-bite Gel in Reducing Mosquito Bite Induced Erythema' by N. Hill et al. Arnica and calendula (and Traumeel S): 'Treatment of Sports Injuries with Traumeel Ointment – a controlled double blind study' by Prof. Dr D. Bohmer and Dr P Ambrus, at the Institute of Sports Medicine Johann Wolfgang Goethe University, Frankfurt, in *Biological Therapy* Vol x, No 4, 1992; 'Therapy Experience with a Homeopathic Ointment: Results of Drug Surveillance Conducted on 3,422 Patients' by Stefan Zenner, *Biological Therapy*, vol XII, No 3, 1994. Rene-Maurice Gattefosse, initial experiment with lavender oil for his own burns, 1930s. Also: antibacterial action: *Pharmazie* no 35, pp 698-701. Aloe Vera: 'Prevention of Ultraviolet Radiation-Induced Suppression of Contact and Delayed Hypersensitivity by Aloe barbadensis Gel Extract' by F. Strickland, R.P. Pelley et al, Dept Immunology, University of Texas/the Anderson Cancer Center, Houston; and University of Texas Medical Branch, Galvaston: in *The Journal of Investigative Dermatology*, 1994.

FLU AND FEVER

Homeopathy: 'A Controlled Evaluation of Homeopathic Preparation in the Treatment of Influenza-like Syndromes' by J.P. Ferley and D. Zmirou, Centre Alpin de Recherche Epidemiologique et de Prevention Sanitaire, Grenoble University Hospital, France, in the *British Journal of Clinical Pharmacology*, 1989, 27; 329-335. Garlic: 'Antimicrobial effects of Allium sativum L. (garlic) Allium Ampeloprasum L. (elephant garlic) and Allium cepa L. (onion), Garlic Compounds and Commercial Garlic Supplement Products' by B.G. Hughes and L.D. Lawson, *Phytotherapy Res.*, 1991, vol 5. Echinacea: 'Adjuvant Immunotherapy with Different Formulations of Echinacin' by E. Coeugniet et al, *Planta Med.* 1994, vol 60; 'Macrophage Activation by the Polysaccharide Arabinogalactan Isolated from Plant Cell Cultures of Echinacea Purpurea' by B. Leuttig et al, *J. Natl. Cancer Institute*, 1989, vol 81; 'The Influence of Immune-stimulating Effects of Repessed Juice from Echinacea Purpurea on the Course and Severity of Colds' by D. Shoenberger, *Forum of Immunology*, 1992, 8: 2-12. Vitamin C: 'The Effect on Winter Illness of Large Doses of Vitamin C' by T.W. Anderson and G. Sduranyyi et al, CMAJ, 1972, vol 111; 'Does Vit C Alleviate the Symptoms of the Common Cold – a review of current evidence' by H. Hemil, in *Scandinavian Journal of Infectious Diseases*, 1994, vol 26.

HEADACHES AND MIGRAINES

Food intolerances/allergies: 'Food Allergy and Adult Migraine' by L.E. Mansfield and T.R. Vaughan et al, *Annals of Allergy*, 1985, vol 55; 'Is Migraine Food Allergy?' J. Egger and C.M. Carter et al, *Lancet* 1985, vol ii; 'Food Allergy in Migraine', J Monro, J. Brostoff et al; *Lancet*, 1980, ii; 'Diet and Migraine: a review of the literature' by J.E. Perkine and J. Harte et al, *Journal of the American Dietetic Association*, 1983, vol 83. Salt: 'Angiotensin and Aldosterone Elevation in Salt-induced Migraine', by J.B. Brainard, *Headache*, 1981, vol 21. Magnesium: 'Magnesium Prophylaxis of Menstrual Migraine' by F. Facchinetti, G. Sances et al, *Headache*, 1991, vol 31. Low protein diets: 'Effect of Carbohydrate-rich Diet, Low in Protein, in Classic and Common Migraine', by L. Hasselmark and R. Malmgren, *Cephalalgia*, 1987, vol 7; 'Effects of Dietary Protein-tryptophan Restriction upon 5-HT Uptake by Platelets and Clinical Symptoms of Migraine-like Headache', *Cephalalgia* 1983, vol 3. Fish oils: High Carbohydrate Diet: 'Dietary Precursors and Brain Transmitter Formation', by J.D. Fernstrom, the *Annual Review of Medicine*, vol 32, 1981. A diet low in tryptophan (one of the major sources of amino acids from which serotonin is made): '*Migraine: a Biochemical Headache*?' by M. Crook, *Biochemistry Society* transcripts, 9 (4), 1981. et al: *The American Journal of Clinical Nutrition*, 1985, vol 41. Magnesium: 'Magnesium and Migraine' by K. Weaver, *Headache*, 1990, 30 (letter); 'Scrum and Salivery Magnesium Levels in Migraine' by V. Gallai, P. Sarchielli et al, *Headache*, 1992, col 32. Calcium and vit. D: 'Vitamin D and Calcium in Menstrual Migraine', by S. Thys-Jacobs, in *Headache* 1994, vol 34. Feverfew: 'Randomised, Double-blind Placebo Controlled Trial of Feverfew in Migraine Prevention' by J.J. Murphy et al, University Hospital, Nottingham, *Lancet*, July 23, 1988; 'Effacacy of Feverfew as a Prophylactic Treatment of Migraine' by E.S. Johnson et al, *The British Medical Journal*, 1985, vol 291. Ginger: 'Ginger in Migraine Headache' by K.C. Srivasta et al, *The Journal of Ethnopharmacology*, 1992, vol 39. Ginko Biloba: 'Inhibition of the Metabolism of Platelet Activating Factor by Three Specific Antagonists from Ginko Biloba', by V Lamant et al, *Biochemical Pharmacology*, 1987, vol 36. Regular eating: 'Insulin-induced Hypoglycemia in Migraine' by J. Pierce, JNNP 34, 1971; 'Effect of Diabetes on Migraine' by J. Blau et al, *Lancet* 2, 241, 1970. Ice cream: 'Ice Cream Headache', J Hulihan, *British Medical Journal*, 1997, 314. White willow: 'Herbal Medicine' by R.F. Weiss, Gothenberg, *Sweden Ab Arcanum*, 1988, vol 31, p 303; *The British Herbal Compendium* ed by P.R. Bradley, vol 1, published by the British Herbal Medicine Association, Dorset, 1992. Homeopathy: 'Homeopathic Treatment of Migraines: a randomised, double blind, controlled study of 60 cases, homeopathic remedy vs placebo', by Bruno Brigo and Giovanni Serpelloni, Verona, Italy; in the *Berlin Journal of Research and Homeopathy*, vol 11, No. 2, March 1991. Acupressure: 'A Controlled Trial of Treatment of Migraine by Acupuncture' by C.A. Vincent, in *The Clinical Journal of Pain* 1989, No. 5; 'Acupuncture vs Metoprolol in Migraine Prophylaxis: a randomised trial of trigger point inactivation' by J. Hesse et al, *Journal of Internal Medicine*, 1994, 235; 'Traditional Chinese Acupuncture for Tension-style Headache: a controlled study' by T. Tavola and C. Gala et al, in *Pain* 1992, vol 48. Milk Thistle for hangovers: 'Randomised Controlled Trial of Silymarin in Patients with Cirrhosis of the Liver' by Ferenci et al, the *Journal of Hepatology*, 9, 1989. Reflexology: *The Journal of Nursing*, June 24, paper by La Fuente, Noguera, Puy et al; at the Institut fur Pflegeforshung, Bern, 1994.

IRRITABLE BOWEL SYNDROME

Chamomile: 'Pharmacological Investigations with Compounds of Chamomile' by U. Achterrath-Tuckerman, R. Kunde et al, *Planta Med.*, 1980, vol 39. Peppermint: 'Peppermint Oil for Irritable Bowel Syndrome: A Multi Centre trial' by M.J. Dew, B.K. Evans et al, in the *British Journal of Clinical Practice*, 1984, vol 38. Peppermint/fennel/wormfood/carraway: 'Phytotherapy in Functional Abdominal Complaints: results of a clinical study of a preparation of several plants' by J. Westphal, M. Horning et al; *Phytomed*, 1996, vol 2. Evening primrose oil: 'Double Blind Crossover Trial of Evening Primrose Oil in Women with Menstrually Related Irritable Bowel Syndrome' by C.J. Cotterell and A.J. Lee, in *Omega-6 Essential Fatty Acids: Pathophysiology and roles in clinical medicine*, 1990, published by Alan Liss, NY. Allergies: 'Food Hypersensitivity in Irritable Bowel Syndrome' by S.J. Bentley and D.J. Pearson, *Lancet*, 1983, ii. Hypnotherapy: 'Individual and Group Hypnotherapy in Treatment of Refractory Irritable Bowel Syndrome' by R.F. Harvey, in *Lancet*, 1989, I. 'Hypnotherapy: Effect on Quality of Life and Economic Consequences of Irritable Bowel Syndrome' by L.A Houghton, D. Heyman and P.J. Whorwell, in *Gut*, 1994; vol 35. Aloe Vera: *Aloe Vera: The Natural Healer* by Paul Honnsey-Pennell, published by Wordsmith, 1995; *The Aloe Vera Handbook*, Max B. Sousen, The Aloe Vera Research Institute, West Valley City, Utah, USA; 'Aloe Vera – Help or Hype?' by Sue Backhouse, in *Gut Reaction* (The Journal of the IBS Network), Summer 1995. Homeopathy: Asa Foetida: 'Asa Foetida bei Colon irritabile' by V.W. Rahlfs und P. Mossinger, *Deutche Medizinische Wschr*, 104, 1978. Homeopathy (general): 'An investigation into the Homeopathic Treatment of Patients with Irritable Bowel Syndrome' by Dr D. Owen, paper presented at the *British Homeopathic Congress*, Feb 1990.

PERIOD PAIN

Black Cohosh: *Out of This Earth – the Essential Handbook of Herbal Medicine*, by Simon Mills, Viking, 1991; *Encyclopaedia of Common Natural Ingredients Used in Foods, Drugs and Cosmetics*, 2 ed. by A.Y Leung and S. Foster, published by John Wiley and Sons, 1996. Homeopathy: sp. belladonna, colocynthis, Dioscorea villosa and Atropinum sulfuricum (as a complex preparation called Spasmofides S: 'Spasomofides S – Ergebnisse einer Anwendungs-beobachtung', by M. Weiser and K. Kusterman, *Biologische Medizin/Heft* 3, Jun 1994. Acupuncture tested in a placebo-controlled, randomised trial: 'Acupuncture for the Treatment of Primary Dysmenorrhea' by J.M. Helms, *Obstetrics and Gynaecology* 1987, 69; 'Pain and Discomfort in Primary Dysmenorrhoea is Reduced by Pre-emptive Acupuncture or Low-frequency TENS', by M. Thomas and T. Lundeberg *European Journal of Physical and Mental Rehabilitation*, 1995, 4; Paper by Olgeson, Flocco et al, in *Obstetrics and Gynaecology* 1993. vol 82 (6).

PID

White Willow (see Arthritis, for research on pain-relieving effects) Vitamin C and Echinacea (see Shingles, Herpes and Cold Sores) for research on immune system-boosting nutrients.

PROSTATITIS

Vitamins A, C, E: '*Biochemical Pharmacology*' by E. Middleton and G. Drzewieki, 1984, vol 33; *Nutritional Medicine* by Dr Stephen Davies and Dr Alan Stewart, Pan,

1987; Zinc: *Urology*, 1976, No. 7 (vol 2); 'Phytotherapy for the Prostate', by Dr A.C. Bush; Dept of Urology, Glasgow Royal Infirmary, in the *British Journal of Urology*, 1996, vol 78.

REPETITIVE STRAIN INJURY

Violin playing: 'Musicians' Playing Related Musculo-skeletal Disorders, an Examination of Risk Factors', by C. Zaza et al, *The American Journal of Industrial Medicine*, 1997, vol 32. D-phenylalanine: 'Use of D-phenylalanine, an Enkephalinase Inhibitor, in the Treatment of Intractable pain', by K. Budd, 1983, *Advances in Pain Res. Therapy* vol 5; L-Tyrptophan: 'The Effects of Dietary Tryptophan on Chronic Maxillofacial Pain and Experimental Pain Tolerance', by S. Seltzer, in *Pain*, 1982, vol 13; 'Pain and Tryptophan', by R.B. King, in the *Journal of Neurosurgery*, 1980, vol 53; 'The Effect of Tryptophan on Post-operative Endodontic Pain', *Oral Surgery, Oral Medicine, Oral Pathology*, 1984 vol 58. Coffee: 'Coffee Contains Potent Opiate Receptor Binding Activity', by J.H. Boublik, *Nature*, 1983, 301. Wintergreen oil: *An Encyclopedia of Common Ingredients Used in Foods*, by A.Y. Leung published by John Wiley and Sons, NY, 1980; *Medical Pharmacology* by A. Goth, published by C.V. Mosby, St Louis, MO 1984, p 367.

SHINGLES, HERPES AND COLD SORES

Colour therapy: 'Alternative Therapies and Simplex Symptoms, *Sphere* (journal of the Herpes Viruses Association), Volume II, issue 2, p 1. Lavender and Tea Tree essential oils: Aroma Science: *The Chemistry and Bioactivity of Essential Oils*, by Dr Maria Lis-Balchin, Amberwood, 1997. L-Lysine: 'Relation of Arginine-lysine Antagonism to Herpes Simplex Growth in Tissue Culture' by R. Griffith et al, 198l, *Chemotherapy*, vol 27; 'A Multicentre Study of Lysine Therapy in Herpes Simplex Infection', by R. Griffith, *Dermatology*, 1978, vol 56. Echinacea: see above in Flu and Fever refs on its anti-viral action. Fidelity and herpes: Hon. Consultant and Snr Lectr, in GU Medicine, at the Middlesex and University College School of Medicine, in *Men's Health Matters* by Nikki Bradford, Vermilion, 1995. Zinc: 'Genital Herpes and Zinc' by J. Fitzherbert, *Medical Journal of Australia*, vol 1, p 399, 1979. White Willow: see Arthritis, (above). Garlic: 'The Antimicrobial Effect of Allinum Sativum (garlic)' by B.G. Hughes and L.D. Lawson, *Phytother Res* 1991, vol 5. Echinacea: 'Macrophage Activation by the Polysaccharide Arabinogalactan Isolated from Plant Cell Cultures of Echinacea Purpurea', by B. Leuttig and C. Steinmuller et al, *J. Natl Cancer Insti* 1989, vol 81.

SORE THROAT

Vit C: 'Does Vitamin C Alleviate the Symptoms of the Common Cold – a review of the current evidence' by H. Hemil et al, *Scandinavian Journal of Infectious Diseases*, 1994, vol 26; 'Vitamin C and the Common Cold: a double blind trial' by T.W. Anderson et al, CMAJ, 1972; 'The Effect on Winter Illness of Large Doses of Vitamin C' by T. Werson and G. Sursnyyi, CMAJ, 1974, 111. Echinacea: 'The Influence of Immune Stimulating Effects of Pressed Juice from Echinacea Purpurea on the Course and Severity of Severe Colds' by D. Schoenberger, *Forum of Immunology*, 1992. Goldenseal: *The British Herbal Compendium*, Vol 1, P.T. Bradley ed, The British Herbal Medicine Association, Bournemouth, 1992, 119-20. Lavender and Tea Tree oil: *Aroma Science* by Dr Maria Lis-Balchin, Amberwood Publishers, 1995; 'Chronic Bronchitis/Sore Throat and Chest: double blind trial' in *Phytotherapy Research* 1989, vol 3; 'Gouttes aux Essences' by J.P. Ferley, N.

Poutignat et al. Homeopathy: 'Untersunchung uber die Behandlung der auten Pharyngitis mit Phytolacca D2', by Von P. Mossinger, *Allgem Homeopath Zeit*, 1976, Sept-Oct; 221 (5).

THRUSH

Acidophilus: 'Ingestion of Yoghurt Containing Lactobascillus as Prophylaxis for Candidal Vaginitis' by E. Hilton and H.D. Isenberg, *Annals of Internal Medicine*, 1992, 116; 'Vaginal Infection' by H. Aschenback, in *Clinical Obstetrics and Gynaecology*, 1983, vol 26; 'Antibacterial Activity Associated with Lactobascillus Acidophilus' by J. Vincent et al, *Journal of Bacteriology*, 1959, vol A78; 'Ingestion of Yogurt Containing Lactobacillus Acidophilus as Prophylaxis for Candidal Vaginitis' by E. Hilton et al, in the *Annals of Internal Medicine*, 1992, vol 116. Aromatherapy: Tea Tree Oil: 'Melaleuca Alterifolia Oil: Uses for Trichomonal Vaginitis and Other Vaginal Infections', by E.O. Pena, in *Obstetrics and Gynaecology*, 1962, vol 19 and *Phytotherapy* No 15, Sept 1985, by Dr Paul Belaiche. Garlic: 'The Antimicrobial Effects of Allium Sativum (garlic)' by B.G. Hughes and L.D. Lawson, in *Phytother Res* 1991, vol 5; Homeopathy: Borax: 'Double Blind Clinical Trial of Borax and Candida in the Treatment of Vaginal Discharge', by Dr Helen Carey *Communications*, Winter 1985.

TOOTHACHE AND TEETHING

Caffeine: 'Ibuprofen Compared with Ibuprofen Plus Caffeine after Third Molar Surgery' by H.J. McQay, *Pain* 1996, vol 66. Vitamin E: 'Endogenous Opiod System in the Realisation of the Analgesic Effect of Alpha Tocopherol' *Biull Eksp Biol Med*, vol 105 (2). Homeopathy complex: 'Zahnungsbeschwerden! Was tun?' Von A.M. Vestweber, *Erfahrungsheilkunde* 3/1994. Arnica and Hypericum: 'Homeopathic Treatment of Dental Neuralgia using Arnica and Hypericum: a summary of 60 observations' by Prof. H. Albertine, William Goldberg et al, in the *Journal of the American Institute of Homeopathy*, 1985, Vol 78, pt 3. Aloe Vera: *The Good Health Guide* frwd. Dr Patrick Pietroni, Bloomsbury, 1984.

VARICOSE VEINS

Homeopathy: 'Complementary Treatment of Varicose Veins – a randomised, placebo-controlled, double blind trial' by E. Ernst et al, *Phlebology*, 1990, 5, 157-63. *The Good Health Guide* frwd. Dr Patrick Pietroni, Bloomsbury, 1984. Bare feet/exercise: Dr Robert May, in *The Medical Tribune*, (Australia) Feb 27, 1980.

THANKS TO

Many grateful thanks to several organisations and companies for the use of their research data bases, and for their advice – especially the NHS Homeopathic Hospital's library in Glasgow, the Royal Society of Medicine, the University of Exeter, Solgar Vitamins, and the Health and Diet Company.